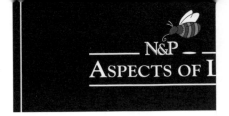

N&P
ASPECTS OF L

Aspects of Life is a series of publications designed to help people respond to the changing circumstances which they face as their lives progress.

In an entertaining and down-to-earth style, the Aspects of Life Series seeks to encourage readers not only to tackle their responsibilities in a more fulfilling way, but also to enjoy the stimulus of new challenges.

The subject matter, which at present ranges through home life, leisure and work, is being chosen to recognise the diversity of experience and opportunities which individuals and families may encounter.

This pioneering venture by a building society draws on N&P's unique experience in responding to customers' requirements, helping people to achieve a better quality of life.

First Published in Great Britain in 1993.

By N&P Publishing, a division of the National & Provincial Building Society, Provincial House, Bradford BD1 1NL, West Yorkshire.

© Maggie Shackleton and Jane Molloy 1993.

Printed and bound in Great Britain by Lund Humphries Limited, Bradford.

Distributed by Book Point Ltd, 39 Milton Park, Abingdon, Oxford OX14 4TD.

Represented by John Wilson Booksellers Ltd, 1 High Street, Princes Risborough, Buckinghamshire HA7 0AG.

British Library cataloguing in publication data record for this title is available from the British Library ISBN number 1 897634 03 X.

The contents of this publication are believed to be correct at time of printing. However, the publishers and authors cannot accept responsibility for errors or omissions, nor for the changes in policy details given. Readers should always satisfy themselves that the facilities they require are available and that prices, where quoted, still apply.

January 1995

To Penny and Andrea,
    We hope that this book won't frighten you but rather give you confidence. Good luck!
        With all our love
            Katie, Chris
                and Amanda.

'When the first baby laughed for the first time, the laugh broke into a thousand pieces and they all went skipping about, and that was the beginning of fairies.'

Peter Pan, JM Barrie. 1860 – 1897

To Betty and Sandy, for bringing us into the world

ACKNOWLEDGMENTS

We would like to thank the following people who helped so much with *Labours of Love*: all the mothers we interviewed – we are sorry we couldn't include you all, but time and space were at a premium; Tony Appi for his help, encouragement and never ending resourcefulness; David Rust for his constant nagging; Sarah Kempton for keeping the children at bay; Hilda Platje for her enormous range of contacts; and Mike Aalders and Mike Molloy for believing in *Labours of Love* and giving us the opportunity to write it.

Maggie Shackleton
Jane Molloy
London, 1993

LABOURS OF LOVE

Women's own experiences of childbirth

MAGGIE SHACKLETON AND JANE MOLLOY

INTRODUCTION

Childbirth is an experience most women share at some stage in their lives. Anyone who is pregnant will be aware of the wealth of literature available on the subject. The majority of these books will describe the biological and factual side of things, and the format of a standard labour. But few will provide the answer to the inevitable question: what is it *really* like?

Until fairly recent times, childbirth was an event that filled people with fear as well as joy. But medical science has made such wonderful advances this century that the possibility of mother and child dying in the labour ward is virtually non-existent. Because fear was part of the ritual for thousands of years, myths, legends and superstitions surrounded the act of childbirth; women withdrew from normal day-to-day society during pregnancy when they would, euphemistically, be referred to as being in 'a delicate condition'.

For the actual birth, only a few privileged specialists would be expected to be present: nurse, doctor, midwife. Only in the last few years has the attendance of the father been accepted, let alone encouraged. Twenty five years ago, the presence of the father was rare; fifty years ago, unthinkable. Apart from a male doctor, the event was strictly a matter of female concern. Even conversations on the subject fell into that category known to men as 'women's talk' and usually brought forth the image of old wives with pursed lips sipping tea while they competed to tell expectant young women of the agonies they'd endured when 'their time had come'. Today the world has changed, thank God.

To find out how much, we talked to women from all walks of life, and the one overriding factor that cannot be ignored is, 'It hurts like hell!' Having said that, it is not something we need be afraid of. Childbirth should be and can be a joyous and fulfilling experience. The more informed we are, the closer we come to that reality. The aim of this book, therefore, is to provide you with a greater insight, by sharing with you other women's accounts of what it was really like for them. Having a baby for the first time is something nobody can adequately describe until they have been through it themselves. While there are similarities, everyone's story is different and everyone will have their own viewpoint on childbirth. Some of you will follow a totally natural path, while others will be happy with the use of pain relief in varying degrees. Whichever route you choose, it should always be the right choice for you as an individual.

The stories in this book have been compiled at random and no attempt has been made to promote any professional school of thought whatsoever. We do not offer you any advice, but wish you to make up your own mind. Hopefully, from each uniquely different story, there will be some valid and useful information that will make the birth of your child a little less mysterious. No matter what your experience, remember that, when you finally hold your child in your arms for the first time, it will all have been worthwhile.

Debbie, 33, independent travel adviser, and Nick, 35, tour manager in the music industry

"The more I thought about the birth the more terrified I became"

"After nine months of 'Oh my God!' I was suddenly very calm"

"I resembled a hot air balloon on legs"

I found out on my 31st birthday, just after a wonderful holiday in Hong Kong, that we'd made a baby. My initial reaction was one of utter terror, first of all knowing how strongly Nick felt against having children and, secondly, knowing how much he enjoyed being a free agent. In all the years we'd been together, we still lived apart, and were really quite independent of each other. I sat outside his house for two hours crying before I finally plucked up the courage to go in and break the news.

Through a lot of tears, I explained the situation, expecting the worst. But completely the opposite reaction came out – he was so delighted. The relief was something else, suddenly I could be proud of myself, 'Wow! I was pregnant', and I felt a great sense of achievement. We decided not to tell anyone for a few months because Nick was going away on tour, and we wanted to be together when we broke the news to our families. Because we weren't married, we were both worried about how they would react.

The week before Nick went away passed in a bit of a blur, but after he'd gone I pretty much pulled myself together. It was just me and the baby now and we'd have to take each day as it came. I went back to work and carried on as normal really. I had no morning sickness, and was beginning to think this was all a bit too easy, when the bombshell dropped.

I was about 12 weeks pregnant, and on my way to Hemel Hempstead visiting a travel agency, when I began to experience the most awful pains in my back and groin. I rang my office to tell them that I wouldn't be back and was halfway up the M1 to my doctor's when the pain got so bad that, for safety's sake, I drove straight on to the Luton and Dunstable hospital. I literally left my engine running in the car park, ran into casualty and said, "Please help me, I think I'm losing my baby".

The staff were absolutely wonderful. I was rushed through immediately and, within minutes, a team of doctors, including the consultant obstetrician, were poring over me. I had all sorts of tests to try to find out what was wrong. They were sure that I wasn't in premature labour, but they didn't know what was causing me to have so much pain. I had scans every day to make sure the baby was okay and they finally discovered that, along with a urinary infection, my left kidney had virtually shut down.

It was all so unreal because I'd never been in hospital in my life, and being on my own and not knowing if I was going to lose the baby absolutely freaked me out. Once we found out what was wrong, however, I was calmer in my mind. Nick was going grey in America, ringing me every day, saying, "I'm coming home, I'm coming home", but I said, "No, I can cope, I'm a soldier". Afterwards, I thought, if we can get through this we can get through anything. I took a month off work and gradually built myself up again. From then on I had no more problems with the pregnancy, except of course getting larger and larger!

The weeks passed and the old emotions went up and down quite a bit. I never knew I could cry quite so much – and at the least little thing. Nick came home and we moved in together, which was lovely, and we decided it was time to let the family in on our little secret. First on the list were Nick's parents. I was really worried about telling them because, as I have said, we weren't married and they are churchgoers with very high morals.

Once again it was the complete opposite of what I had expected. All this love just poured out of them and it was very emotional. This was on the Friday, and on the Saturday we packed our bags and headed off to see my parents in Cornwall. I'd bottled it up for so long I couldn't get there fast enough.

We arrived and the initial reaction was one of confusion: "What are you doing here, something's wrong?" We both laughed and I casually said, "What are you doing the first week in January?" Daddy was sitting there with this very old-fashioned look on his face and asked, "Why?" Nick was hanging on to me for grim death and I just blurted out, "You are going to be grandparents". There was about three

4

seconds of silence and then about 20 seconds of "Whaa!" Within half an hour there were about 30 of us in the 'Farmers Arms' and the Champagne was flowing.

A few weeks later Nick was offered a world tour with the B-52s, too good an offer to turn down. Although it meant I'd be alone for the rest of my pregnancy, it didn't really worry me, and anyway we needed the money so there wasn't much I could do about it. By October I had to give up work because I was just so tired. It was a long drive there and back and I couldn't manage it any more.

When Nick got home in November I was seven and a half months pregnant… and huge. I think he got a bit of a shock! It really hit him that he was going to be a Dad. He'd been away for so long, he'd switched off emotionally in order to be able to get on with the job, and now suddenly it all sank in. We both realised at this point that it wasn't just the two of us any more, we were going to be a family.

I didn't really have a birth plan, I just wanted to wait and see what happened. The more I thought about the birth the more terrified I became, and wondered what my pain threshold would be. In the end I decided to rely on instinct and to let my body decide when and if it needed pain relief.

My sister, Vicky, arrived to spend Christmas with us and give me a hand because by now I resembled a hot air balloon on legs. I couldn't get comfortable, I couldn't eat, I couldn't do anything. Then, on 28th December, I had my show. At first I just had bad period-type pains and then after a while they got quite regular. I thought, 'Wow, this is it', and we were all running around in a bit of a panic, but then they died off again, and it was pretty much the same for the rest of the day. None of us got much sleep that night; I can't say I was in pain, but I kept getting these funny sort of twinges.

All day Sunday I still had dull sort of period pains but worst of all was the backache. We decided to call the community midwife as we weren't really sure what was happening, and she came over to examine me. She explained that, although I hadn't begun to dilate, things were definitely moving and I was in the early stages of labour. I was told to stay at home for as long as possible because with the New Year approaching the hospital was under-staffed and therefore very busy. Nick joked that it was typical of me to give birth just when everybody was out partying.

For the rest of the day the contractions were very weak, there was one every hour, then one every half hour. They were very inconsistent and in my mind I knew I wasn't ready yet. Monday came and the day progressed pretty much the same as Sunday. That evening Vicky said, "Look, I'll stay up with Debbie, Nick. You go and get some sleep". It was about 11.30 – Nick hadn't been in bed more than half an hour – when the contractions started to come more frequently. The pain was intensifying all the time and Vicky fetched the Tens machine that we had hired a few weeks earlier.

I put it on very low, but it didn't seem to help much. We tried to watch some telly, but typically there was nothing worth watching. I kept getting up and walking around from room to room; I tried to do some ironing, made four million cups of coffee, but nothing helped to settle me. I suddenly got a terrible attack of claustrophobia, I just had to get out of the house. It was 1.30 in the morning and I said to Vicky, "Come on, I can't stand this. Let's go for a walk". So, Tens machine and all, off we go.

Every 100 yards I was hanging on to the wall or someone's gate; the pain was definitely hotting up by now. Vicky suddenly spied an abandoned shopping trolley and, jumping in, said, "Come on Debbie, now's your chance to get some practise in". So there I was in full labour having absolute hysterics wheeling my nutty sister down the middle of the road. God knows what we must have looked liked, but it certainly helped me to relax!

We were just opening the front door when I got the most almightiest contraction. I remember saying, "Whoa… that was a serious one". They were coming every ten minutes and at 2.15 I sent Vicky up to wake Nick. I'll never forget him running down the stairs, still half asleep, shouting, "What sandwiches do you want?" Not let's get you to the hospital but what sandwiches do you want! It was really weird because after nine months of 'Oh my God!' I was suddenly very calm. As we got in the car I was expecting Nick to do a Nigel Mansell. Throughout the pregnancy we'd both had this image of a fast and furious drive to the hospital, but instead we drove really slowly. There was a great sense of tranquillity and neither of us were in a panic. The pain was bad but I just kept thinking, 'Millions of women have been through this, so let's have no fuss' and, as we arrived, Nick rang the night bell and very calmly said, "Hello, we're going to have our baby".

They took me to the delivery room and as I got undressed I was holding on to my stomach thinking, 'Any minute now everything's going to fall out!' The midwife came to examine me and I'll never forget those wonderful words of hers: "My dear, you're 5cms dilated, you've done most of the work on your own". I was absolutely thrilled to bits, you know, you feel like you've just climbed Mount Everest or something. She asked me if I wanted my waters broken, and I know this sounds silly, but despite all the years I'd been with Nick I really didn't want him to see it happen. I explained how I felt and he said, "Look don't be so daft". Suddenly I realised that she was right, there I was with my legs akimbo and all my worldly goods on show, and I'd been worried about a silly thing like that.

As they were broken I felt this incredible whoosh as all this hot liquid ran down my legs. Oh the relief! Within a split second I had a terrible urge to push, but it was too quick and I was told not to give in to it. The midwife gave me some gas and air and I remember focusing on this crabby old picture on the wall. The nurse said, "I'm going to leave you on your own, everything's perfectly all right", and off she went. Nick had made up some tapes of all our romantic favourites and we put one on.

The pain was dreadful, it was a pain I'd never experienced before, so I didn't know whether it would get worse or stay the same. The contractions were coming every two minutes and lasting about 30 seconds; I was coping with them as best I could. The gas and air really did help although it made me feel high as a kite, giggling, and completely spaced out. Nick was taking as much as I was and soon we were having our own private party.

Things got a bit out of hand when the midwife walked in and I said, "Oh God, here comes Doctor Crippin!" We were soon brought back down to earth when she informed us that I was fully dilated and could start pushing. I looked up at the clock, it was 6am, and I remember thinking, 'Any minute now I'm going to have my baby'. I was surprised at how much hard work the pushing was, and not having had any sleep for the last three days didn't help matters. I was beginning to get exhausted. When they told me that I was fully dilated I expected the baby to be born fairly quickly but this stage seemed to be going on and on. I was pushing and pushing. Nick and the midwife were trying to calm me down, telling me that they could see the head crowning… and then it started to burn.

I grabbed hold of Nick and screamed, "I can't carry on, it's hurting too much". Nick suddenly took complete control and said, "Look, she's had enough, she's been trying to push this baby out for hours. Can't you do something to help her?" The doctor was called and I was removed to a much larger delivery suite where they prepared to do a ventouse extraction (where they use a suction cap). My legs were put up in stirrups and I was given an episiotomy, which I didn't feel at all. The doctor attached the ventouse to the baby's head and told me to push, which isn't easy when your legs are at 45 degree angles. I remember giving one almighty push that felt like somebody had set fire to me down there and then the next thing I knew Nick was saying, "Oh my God it's a baby. Debbie look, we've got a son".

I just filled up with emotion, the tears were streaming down my cheeks and I felt like the only person in the world to have given birth, so absolutely special. It was New Year's Eve and they wouldn't let the dads stay to see the New Year in. As Nick left he gave me two cards which I wasn't allowed to open until midnight. As 12 o'clock approached I began to feel really alone and sad. We should have been together as a family celebrating.

I cracked open my little bottle of Lucozade and reached for the cards that Nick had left me. One was to Jordon and said, 'To my Son, welcome to the World from your Father', and the other was to thank me for making it possible. I took Jordon in my arms and suddenly felt like the happiest person alive.

Shelly, 31, skills and management development consultant, and Peter, 32, lecturer

"I'm not going to make it to the hospital, I'm not even going to make it to the front door"

"Call the doctor, this baby is going to be born here and be born now!"

"I screamed 'Get that cat out of here' and with the next push my baby was born"

Kara was three and half when I found myself pregnant again. Peter and I had planned to have a second child around about this time, so it was great, absolutely what we wanted. Then, disaster. A week later Peter was made redundant. We were in the middle of doing up the house: that all had to stop and there was no other alternative than for me to carry on working. I am a consultant to the Police on race relations and equal opportunities, so I was having to commute to the training school in Bedford, which is a 135-mile round trip.

It was a real slog, but luckily the pregnancy ticked along nicely, although I have to admit to being very tired with all the travelling. The course finished on the Monday, which was great because according to the hospital dates my baby was due the following Friday. My mother had just arrived from Barbados, and on the Tuesday evening we all sat around having supper and discussing the arrival of the new baby. Peter had an important meeting the next day and said, "Well, whatever you do Shelly, don't have it tomorrow".

The following morning I woke up at about 7.30, desperate to go to the loo. I went to the bathroom, and had just got back into bed again when I heard this tiny sound, like a little 'pop', and thought, 'What was that?' I immediately needed to go to the loo again. When I got there I actually poured and I said to Peter, "This is either the longest wee in history or my waters have just broken". After the conversation last night at supper he thought I was joking and it took a moment or two to persuade him I wasn't.

Neither of us were quite sure what to do next. My waters had broken with Kara on the Monday, but she hadn't been born until the Tuesday, so I wasn't expecting anything to happen straight away. However, Kara had been a breech birth and because of that I knew I ought to get to hospital fairly quickly. I called my GP and explained that I had no pain, just that my waters had broken. She said that as second babies can come quite quickly, I ought to make my way to the hospital fairly soon. This was about 7.40 and Peter and I were trying to work out what to do about his meeting, when at 8.10 I had my first contraction. It was quite strong and I was concerned about getting Kara to school, so I rang my friend and asked her if she could come and pick her up. My Mum was still asleep, which was good because she would only have panicked, you know what mums are like, and that was the last thing I needed. My next contraction was stronger and I thought I'd better time them. I got it completely the wrong way round, though, and timed the actual length of the contraction instead of the space in between – oh, the stupid things you do! Anyway, I eventually worked out that they were coming every three minutes and the bursts of pain were excruciating, but somehow manageable.

With Kara's birth the contractions had been coming every three minutes but then tailed off again, so I thought, 'I'll take the time to get myself together'. I was walking around the bedroom trying to get everything packed and Peter was in the bathroom. I kept going to him and saying, "Well, this is every three minutes". I had three at three minutes, then three at two minutes, and by now it was 8.20am. I was trying to picture the journey to the hospital, my back was hurting and all I wanted to do was lie down and have Peter rub it.

The pain was becoming overwhelming and I was starting to get worried. I threw on some clothes and tried to make my way downstairs. I caught a glimpse of myself in the bathroom mirror and had quite a shock. I looked absolutely ashen and my face was literally dripping. At that point I realised I was in full labour: this was not preparation, this was it.

I couldn't get down the stairs. I kept thinking, 'Will I be able to catch my breath?' I waited, but I just couldn't, the contractions were coming too fast. Somehow I managed to get to the bottom. By now it was 8.45, my Mum was awake and panicking. Both she and Peter were rushing around putting bags in the car. I asked them to call the doctor, but Peter said, "No, you are just panicking, get in the car and we'll get you to hospital".

My daughter Kara was crying because she could see how much pain I was in, and eventually I hit the stairs really hard with my hand and yelled at them, "Call the doctor *now*, this baby is going to be born here and be born *now!*" Thankfully, at that moment my friend Annie arrived to take Kara to school. She took one look at me and said, "Shelly, are you okay?" and I said, "No, I want to push *now!*"

Annie looked at Peter and I think he suddenly realised the seriousness of the situation and finally called the doctor. I called after Kara as she left, "Don't worry darling, Mummy's all right", which was true because by now I felt quite controlled. I knew what was happening and it was all very clear. The doctor arrived within five minutes and I could hear her saying, "Well, I've called an ambulance and she'll probably make it to the local hospital".

I almost screamed at them, "I'm not going to make it to the hospital, I'm not even going to make it out of the front door". The doctor suddenly took control of the situation and said, "Okay, let's find somewhere where you can have the baby. How about the sitting room floor?" It was funny, because my first thought was, 'Oh, no you don't, I've just had the carpet cleaned'. I suggested instead, "How about the kitchen floor?"

Peter rushed off to get the bean bag, blankets and sheets. I was desperately trying to breathe through the pain and then I seemed to get a moment's respite which enabled me to crawl, literally, from the bottom of the stairs to the kitchen. Then the midwives arrived.

I don't know when they'd been called but I was pretty glad to see them. They wanted to examine me and I said, "Listen, don't touch me". I was actually very rude but I didn't care.

They tried to persuade me again and I said, "Look I've told you, don't touch me, the baby is coming, just deliver it". My Mum tried to mediate but I just wanted to be left alone. I knew I had work to do and I needed to concentrate.

At that moment, about 9.30, my friend Ruth, who is also a midwife, arrived because she'd heard on the grapevine what was happening. She was great and told me to do whatever I wanted. I said, "I just want to push" and she said, "Okay, let's go". Quite frankly, I had been trying to hold back. I must have been fully dilated when I was sitting at the bottom of the stairs. It was such a relief, at long last, to be given the go-ahead to start pushing.

Peter was holding my hand and asking whether I was fully dilated when the midwife said, "Well, here's the head, so I guess she must be". She put some towels underneath me when suddenly the cat leapt in through the catflap and promptly trotted over them. I screamed, "Get that cat out of here", and with the next push the baby was born. It had all happened so fast, the doctor had arrived at 9.25, the midwives at 9.30 and my son at 9.35. Great scenes of celebration followed. My Mum and Peter were hugging each other. The doctor was patting the midwives on the back, the midwives were patting the doctor on the back and I was lying there thinking: 'I've just had a baby, with no pain-killers, no gas and air and on my kitchen floor'. I would never have believed it possible.

Sue, 33, career in marketing, and has just completed an Open University degree in psychology, and Nigel, 35, stockbroker

"I was in labour and I was only 28 weeks and one day pregnant"

"I'd waited seven years to have this baby and I wanted it to be the happiest day of my life"

"I haven't done my antenatal classes, I don't know what to do"

I'd sort of given up the whole idea of getting pregnant. We had been trying for seven years and nothing had happened, so when it finally did, well, it was a miracle. We were so utterly delighted that for days we could hardly believe it: after all that time, it was a dream come true.

I had no problems whatsoever. I rarely felt sick, I didn't seem to suffer from tiredness as some women do and generally life carried on as normal – which was a Godsend because in my third month we moved into a new house. As you can imagine it was totally hectic, we were surrounded by packing crates, workmen, dust, you name it, and to have felt lousy all the time would have been a nightmare.

I was 28 weeks pregnant when I heard on the radio as I drove to work that there had been a terrible train crash near Clapham. I completely freaked out because it was very possible that my husband was on one of the trains involved. My heart was pounding as I tried to get through the rush hour traffic, I just wanted to get to a phone and find out if he was all right. By the time I reached the office I was in a terrible state and although it turned out that my husband was okay, one of my colleagues discovered that her son actually was on one of the trains, so it was a pretty traumatic morning.

I carried on with my work as best I could and I suppose it must have been about mid-morning when suddenly, to put it bluntly, I felt as though I'd wet myself. It really surprised me and I genuinely thought that the baby had moved on to my bladder or something. I wasn't in the slightest bit worried and didn't give it a second thought.

With all the chaos of the day I was really relieved to get home. I put the kettle on and rang my best friend to tell her all about the day's events. I was saying goodbye when I remembered peeing myself and I jokingly told her, "Oh yes, and to top it all I've become incontinent". She seemed to think that I should ring my doctor and I really wasn't going to, I thought it was nothing. However, her reaction nagged me, so in the end I did. The doctor advised me to go along to the hospital and said, "You had better pack a toothbrush". I literally did what he said and threw a toothbrush into my handbag. I mean, what's the use of just a toothbrush. I must have been going through a ridiculous phase!

So me and my toothbrush set off for the hospital, the traffic was awful, and I was cursing and swearing. I found the whole thing such an inconvenience, I wasn't worried in the slightest. Anyway, I got there and, by chance, walking down the corridor towards me was a gynaecologist, Mr Worth, who had treated me in the past for a positive smear test. He recognised me immediately and asked what I was doing there. I explained the situation and he took complete control.

I was whisked up to the antenatal ward and after an examination was told that my 'behind' waters had broken. Apparently there are two sets of waters which can break independently of each other. The behind waters are small and there isn't much liquid, unlike the fore waters which usually gush everywhere. Mr Worth then explained that I would have to stay in bed until the baby was born. I was completely flabbergasted, it was 12th December and my baby wasn't due until 1st March.

I can remember thinking, 'He must be mad' and said, "I can't stay in bed until then!" But he was adamant, because once your waters break you are open to infection and they can't take the added risk of premature labour. I hadn't even told my husband that I had gone to the hospital, and he had gone out for a drink straight after work so I hadn't been able to contact him. I had left several frantic messages on the answering machine and poor Nigel arrived home to an empty house and discovered them all: there were also other messages from the friend I'd spoken to earlier wanting to know what the doctor had said. By the time Nigel arrived, I was completely hysterical, not because I was frightened, but because I couldn't imagine staying in hospital for the next three months, not even being allowed out of bed to go to the toilet. I still had all my baby shopping to do and nothing was organised. Nigel was really sweet and said he would do everything, but I still hardly slept that night and woke up feeling just as frustrated. Around lunchtime I started to get terrible backache and just couldn't get myself comfortable. I tried lots of different positions and lots of cushions but nothing seemed to work. I couldn't keep myself still; there I was shuffling around in the bed every 30 seconds when I was supposed to be getting some rest. The bedpans were awful and I couldn't get used to them.

By the afternoon I was so fed up I snuck out of bed to go to the loo and to my horror discovered that I had a show. I told the medical staff and all hell let loose. I was in labour and only 28 weeks and one day into my pregnancy. Oh my God!

I felt like I was on another planet, looking down on myself, I couldn't quite take it in. There was no fear, just complete bewilderment. Mr Worth arrived immediately and I was told that I would have to be moved to another hospital where there was an incubator available. I was hooked up to a drip, which supposedly slows everything down and can sometimes halt labour altogether. They were hoping that they could stop the labour progressing any further, at least until I reached the new hospital. In fact, sometimes it can prevent women from giving birth for weeks; as long as the baby is still getting nourishment from the placenta it's the best way possible.

I don't know what was in the drip but it was as if pure alcohol had been pumped into me. The sensation was appalling, like I'd had masses to drink; the room was spinning and I felt like I wanted to throw up. After an hour on the phone an incubator was located at Tooting and a 999 call was put out for an ambulance. I had no idea exactly how desperate the quest for an incubator is. People have to travel from one end of the country to another just to find adequate facilities.

I was beginning to get frightened by now, Nigel hadn't arrived and they were insisting that we leave immediately. I wasn't prepared to go anywhere without him and I was being taken forcibly into the ambulance when luckily he arrived. We took off at breakneck speed to Tooting through the Wandsworth one-way system the wrong way round. It was right in the middle of the rush hour and it was the only way the driver could get past all the traffic – much to Nigel's excitement.

We arrived at St George's where I was immediately taken for a scan. The results showed that the baby was under 2lbs, and it was at this point that the full implications of my situation were explained to me. I was told that a baby of this size might live, probably would live, but I would have to really prepare myself for the fact that it could be mentally or physically handicapped.

Now I was worried, really worried, but I didn't panic or lose control. It was all a jumble in my mind, I just wanted the baby to be born and not be handicapped. It never for one minute entered my head that the baby might die. If I'd let thoughts like that overtake me I wouldn't have been able to handle it. I'd waited seven years to have this baby and if I was about to give birth I wanted it to be the happiest day of my life, no matter what the outcome.

Nigel and I were taken to a labour room and, because the drip had slowed everything down, my contractions weren't very painful and it was suggested that we both try and get some sleep. Everybody was hopeful that the drip would succeed in stopping the labour altogether. I remember that little room so clearly and as I lay there counting the cracks in the ceiling I said several prayers before finally drifting off to sleep.

I awoke with a start the next morning and after several seconds realised why. Far from slowing down, the contractions had intensified and were now coming thick and fast. We rang the bell and were instantly swamped by midwives, doctors and even the odd professor. As they examined me, I begged them to take the drip off, it obviously wasn't working; and it was confirmed that I was in labour, there was no going back and I would have to go through the normal birth process.

I remember saying to Nigel, "I haven't done my antenatal classes, I don't know what to do". I should have had 11 more weeks to prepare for this moment and I really began to panic. Nigel was brilliant, he said, "Oh, I know what to do. You count to five and then take in a big breath and blow". I don't know why I believed him, he's a stockbroker for goodness sake, but there I was doing everything he said. I've since found out it's nothing like that at all, but we were both doing it together and he was so convincing that it really helped me.

It was around ten in the morning now and the contractions were getting faster and more painful. They asked me what sort of painkiller

I wanted and ran through the list: "Tens, epidural, gas and air". I vaguely remembered a friend saying gas and air was quite good, so I decided on that.

My Mum arrived, which was great because she was very calm and chatted on as if everything was completely normal. I remember her holding my hand which still had the needle attached to it from where the drip had been, and each time I got a contraction she would squeeze it. I don't know which was more painful, the contraction or the pain in my hand. It didn't seem to matter how often I told her to stop, she just kept forgetting.

At about elevenish they examined me again and said I was 5cms dilated and that it would be a long day. Mummy suggested that Nigel, who was looking very dishevelled indeed after spending the night on a bean bag, should go and have a shower, so that at least one of us would be feeling fresher. Off he went to the bathroom, which was down the corridor.

Suddenly the contractions began to get faster and faster and I said to Mummy, "How do you know when the baby is coming?" and she said to me, "Well darling, it's a very similar feeling to wanting to go to the toilet, if you know what I mean?" That's exactly the feeling I was having and luckily there was a nurse walking past so I called her in and asked her the same thing. She examined me, looked up, and said, "It's coming!"

Then there was real panic. People were running everywhere and I could hear the alarm bell which alerts the special care baby unit that a baby is on its way. They told me to lie on my side, hold my legs together and whatever happened not to push, which was extremely difficult because the urge was engulfing me.

Mummy ran off to get Nigel, and we laugh about it now, because there he was, happily in the middle of his shower, when he heard my mother shouting, "Nigel come quickly, the baby is being born". He literally jumped out of the shower, tore down the corridor and presented himself, completely naked and dripping wet. It really was a farcical scene. Mummy was shouting at him to put some clothes on and poor Nigel didn't know whether he was coming or going.

There was so much going on that I didn't have time to contemplate what was happening. There seemed to be hundreds of people all working away frantically. They performed a complete episiotomy to ensure an unobstructed delivery. At only 28 weeks premature babies' heads are so soft and tiny that they can easily be damaged.

The pain was excruciating and I can't honestly tell you which hurt most, the cut or the contractions, because it all seemed to mingle into one. I was hanging on to the gas and air for dear life when suddenly I became aware of Nigel trying to pull it away from me. Somewhere in the confusion I heard a voice saying, "Take the gas and air away, she's got to concentrate on pushing".

I remember not wanting to let go, it was the only thing that seemed to be helping me. Nigel and I were having a real battle over the gas and air, my Mum was still squeezing my hand. God, I'll never forget her squeezing that hand and it hurting as well as all the rest of it.

At this point there seemed to be a rush of voices from all directions telling me what to do, including my Mother. I didn't know what was going on: should I be pushing, holding back or what? I was frightened, because it was all happening so fast and I didn't feel as if I was in control of anything; in fact, I was totally out of control.

I yelled out, "Will you please all shut up and just one of you tell me what to do". It was brilliant, an Irish doctor with a great booming voice came forward and I just focused on him. I wanted so much for the birth to be over with now. I definitely had this image in my head of a deformed baby and the suspense and tension of the past few hours was exhausting me. I needed to know now what the outcome was, good or bad.

With three pushes she was born and all I saw was just masses of black hair and something so unbelievably tiny. I wanted to touch her, to look at her, but of course you can't, and they whisked her away instantly. I could hear the doctors saying, "She looks all right, she seems okay", and a cheer went up as she weighed in at nearly 3lbs. Her weight was good and she was breathing on her own; the relief in the room was enormous.

Everybody was overjoyed and suddenly I found myself relaxing. I remember being really, really happy, I felt chuffed, I suppose like any other woman who has just had a baby. While they began to stitch me up, Nigel went off to ring everybody with the good news. And it *was* good news because, no matter what the outcome, we'd had a baby girl and we felt enormously proud.

As soon as I was physically able I went down to see her. It was a scary moment. She looked like a little rat, covered in foetal hair, she was so tiny, her legs were so skinny and the skin hung off her bones like an old person. Her eyes were gigantic because they were all out of proportion to the rest of her. But to us she was lovely. Nigel kept on saying, "Isn't she beautiful, isn't she beautiful". They told me I could stroke her, but I wasn't brave enough. There were millions and millions of monitors, she was on a drip and I remember the tube was bigger than her whole arm, and what if I jogged her and the needle moved?

It wasn't until the middle of the night that I got really tearful: everybody had gone home and I found myself alone. I wanted to go down to see her and that's when I held her for the first time. I was scared stiff, but it was lovely, and from that moment on I became obsessed with the fact that she would get stronger if I was holding her. I don't know if you call it God or what, but suddenly I just knew that everything would be all right.

Eight weeks later, weighing in at 5lbs, Katherine came home for the first time. She is now a healthy, bouncy four-year-old and has suffered no ill effects from her early entrance into the World.

Carmel, 29, secretary, and now a full-time mother, and Steve, 33, building contractor

"Oh my God, they're cutting me open"

"I'll never look at *Top of the Pops* in the same light again"

"I had a 'show' every day and every day I thought, 'This is it'"

I'd only been married eight weeks when I found out I was pregnant. It was quite a shock because I'd always had this nagging doubt that I wouldn't be able to conceive – I think a lot of people have that – so I was really delighted and proud of myself. Although I had done a pregnancy test just before Christmas, which had showed up negative, I *felt* different, my back ached and my boobs kept tingling. I told my Mother and she said, "Sounds to me like you're pregnant, why don't you do another test?" This time it was positive and from the way I was feeling I knew for certain that I was.

I rang my husband at work which I normally don't do because he's always so busy. He was quite short with me and said, "Well, is it important?" I thought, 'Oh God, I don't want to tell him now', but I blurted it out anyway. Obviously he was really pleased and we just sort of took it from there.

When I got to about eight or nine weeks I was being sick all the time, sometimes as often as three times a day, and I was like that literally right up until I had the baby. I worried about it a lot, but the hospital reassured me that it couldn't harm the baby in any way, and I suppose in the end I got used to it. Being sick didn't stop me from eating though. We'd go out for a meal at least three or four times a week. The guys at the local Indian restaurant used to joke with Steve that if I wasn't careful I'd end up giving birth in front of all their customers.

I found I cried a lot and over the most ridiculous things. Steve would say something quite innocuous to me and I'd bawl my head off; he couldn't believe it. I wasn't depressed or anything, I just couldn't stop crying!

I'm confused as to whether or not I enjoyed being pregnant, because at the time I grumbled incessantly about being overweight and feeling awkward. My chest was enormous, it was just dreadful, I felt like Dolly Parton. Looking back, though, I get quite nostalgic and wonder whether it was really quite as bad as I made out.

For a long time the baby was in a breech position and I was told that if it didn't turn I'd probably end up having a Caesarean. I wasn't too bothered by this, I didn't think I had a very high pain threshold anyway and right from the start thought I'd plump for the epidural. Anyway, at 34 weeks the baby did turn, and in some ways I was a bit peeved. You get used to one idea and now I had to start thinking differently. Steve was the most encouraging; he told me to think positively and not to worry, just see how things progressed when the time came.

The baby was due on 6th September and the week before that I fell over. We'd decided to go for a walk in the park and I was waiting on the doorstep for Steve to put his trainers on. Maybe it was because I was so big and cumbersome, I really don't know, but somehow I lost my balance and fell straight into the hedge. I sprained my ankle badly and was terrified something might have happened to the baby.

We sent for the doctor, who seemed to think that everything was fine, except that she hadn't brought along her little trumpet thing to listen to the baby's heartbeat and thought it best that we go to hospital for a proper check. I was in a complete panic now, the doctor kept saying, "Don't worry", but that's easier said than done. It wasn't until I was wired up to the foetal heart monitor and could actually hear the rhythmic beating that I began to relax. I stayed there for ages, it was such a reassuring sound.

The following Friday I was booked in for an ultrasound and told that the baby was really big, at least eight-and-a-half to nine pounds. I was flabbergasted; how was I going to get it out? My eyes watered at the thought. I kept thinking, 'If only it had remained breech I could have had a Caesarean', because that was far more preferable to pushing out a nine-pounder. For the last couple of weeks I'd been experiencing Braxtons Hicks contractions which were quite painful at times and I was really fed up with the whole thing. The 6th came and went and nothing had happened, so when people rang up asking, "Have you had it yet?" I felt like saying, "Well, if I had I wouldn't be sitting here at home".

I was a week overdue when I went for my last hospital appointment and told the midwife about the pains I'd been having. She decided to give me an internal examination and found that I was already 1cm dilated. I thought, 'Great, I've done 1cm already and it didn't really hurt that much, so the rest can't be that bad'. Although the head hadn't engaged yet she seemed pretty certain that I'd have the baby over the weekend. I went home on a high, thinking, 'Any minute now'.

All weekend I was in a fluster every time I got even the faintest twinge. Then on Sunday I had a show. 'This is it,' I thought, but other than the usual pains I'd been having all along, nothing happened.

By Monday morning I was beginning to think I'd be stuck with this lump forever. Late that afternoon I had another show. This time I rang the hospital because I wasn't sure whether this was right or not. It was only a slight spotting and I was told it was perfectly normal: "Don't worry, baby will be here soon". But still nothing happened. I had a show every day and every day I thought, 'This is it'.

By the time Thursday came I was so fed up I decided to go for a walk. It was a lovely warm autumn day, but just getting to the end of the road seemed like such an effort and after only ten minutes I had to turn back. I got home and lay down on the bed. I was exhausted. My baby was now 11 days late; nearly three weeks ago they had told me it was nearly 9lbs; and, lying there looking at my stomach, I was convinced it was now more like 19. Just at that moment I felt a warm rush of water, there wasn't much liquid, so I wasn't sure if my waters had broken or not. I rang the hospital and was told to come in straight away. Finally, after all the false hopes, this *was* it.

Steve was working on the other side of town and it took him quite a while to get home. He probably thought it would all progress really slowly and that I'd just be having the odd contraction. In fact, they were coming very fast indeed, near enough every four minutes, and the pain took my breath away.

I was quite frightened, this wasn't supposed to be happening so fast. According to the books I'd read, you should get one every 10 to 15 minutes to start with. I went downstairs and got my bag ready and decided to clear up the kitchen. Everybody would be coming back to see Steve after the birth and I didn't want them to find the place in a mess. More than anything it was helping to take my mind off the pain.

23

When Steve eventually got home he decided to have a shower and change because we anticipated a long night. I was calm, but when the pain became intense I think I did panic, and then I just wanted to get to the hospital for some pain relief. We got in the car and Steve drove right to the top of the road before turning round. It only put about one minute on the journey but I was fuming, that was one vital minute to me, things were happening so fast I just wanted to get there. I remember gripping my hands on the dashboard and taking deep breaths.

Steve managed to park the car quite close to the entrance which I was really relieved about because I didn't think I could walk too far. By now it was about 6.30 in the evening, and I was immediately taken to a delivery suite where they examined me. I was only about 2cms dilated by then which really depressed me. I thought, 'This pain is very intense and if I'm only 2cms dilated God only knows what the rest of it's going to be like'.

They attached me to the foetal heart monitor and placed another one on my stomach so they could chart my contractions. I was clutching the sides of the bed and moaning that it hurt so much. One of the midwives said, "You know, on the Richter scale of things that wasn't really a big one". Steve was telling me to be calm, to try and get through the pain barrier, and I thought, 'God, I wish you were going through this instead of me'. They wheeled in a TV set and *Top of the Pops* was on. I remember thinking, 'I'll never look at *Top of the Pops* in the same light again'.

I wasn't coping with the pain at all well and I asked the midwife to give me something. She suggested I had some Pethidine and I really thought it would ease the pain totally but, honestly, it did absolutely nothing for me. They come at you with this big injection and you think it will work wonders but all it does is make you a bit dopey.

The pain was just getting worse and worse so the next time the midwife came in I asked for the epidural. I was expecting to get it straight away but of course the anaesthetist was busy with other people. This is one of the things you're not aware of when you go into labour: apparently it's very common to be begging for the epidural and having to wait up to an hour and a half for it.

When he finally arrived at 9pm I told him that if possible I still wanted to have some movement in my legs. He said, "That's not a problem.

I'll give you a mobile epidural which will numb only your pelvic area". Within minutes I felt like a normal person again, much more in control.

I got up and they helped me walk over to a rocking chair in front of the TV where I sat thinking, 'My God, I can't believe I'm in labour, this is wonderful and so relaxing'. I could still feel the contractions but it was more like a movement than real pain. I could see them rising and falling on the monitor and Steve was saying, "Wow! that was a big one". I was just so delighted I hadn't felt it.

I thought, 'Well, this is great, I'll stay in the chair until I'm 10cms dilated and then I'll just pop up on to the bed and give birth'. I noticed that the midwife kept looking at the monitor screen and I asked if everything was okay. I could see for myself that each time I had a contraction the baby's heartbeat dipped. She said, "There's nothing to worry about but I'm just going to get the senior midwife to come and have a look". I thought, 'Hold on a minute, there's something wrong here'.

They explained that they were sure the baby wasn't in distress but were concerned that it might not be getting enough oxygen. Well, that was it. I kept imagining brain damage or something. They gave me the oxygen mask and suddenly it was all a bit more medical, which frightened me even more.

Over the next ten minutes things didn't improve and a consultant was called in. He took a look at the chart and decided they were going to take some blood from the baby's head, to make sure it was getting enough oxygen. They were very calm and kept reassuring me that everything was still quite normal, but it didn't sound very normal to me.

The results were back within minutes and the baby was fine. Steve and I breathed a sigh of relief and I told him to go off and ring my Mum to let her know that everything was going okay. I couldn't take my eyes off the monitor. The midwife turned the screen away from me as she thought I was getting too upset, but I could still hear it. On my next contraction the heartbeat really dipped and I shouted to the midwife, "It's getting weaker isn't it?" She said, "Yes, I'm quite concerned about it now. I'm just going to press this button here to call another doctor". I now realise that she hit the emergency button, because three doctors and a paediatrician came flying in.

Poor Steve came back to find the room full of people. The consultant explained that they were very concerned about the baby's heartbeat; it was dipping far more than they would have liked and they were going to do another blood test. The doctor took one look at the results and said, "I'm sorry, the baby's oxygen is too low, we're going to have to do an immediate Caesarean".

The papers were brought for me to sign – it's quite scary really, like signing your life away – and I was wheeled down to the operating theatre. The journey there seemed to take forever and all I could think was, 'Get my baby out, what if its heart has already stopped and they don't know'.

They lifted me on to the operating table; I remember seeing these enormous lights and everybody masked up, even Steve. They gave me another epidural which completely numbed my legs so I couldn't feel a thing. There was some music playing and Steve said, "Just concentrate on the music" but I kept thinking, 'Oh my God, they're cutting me open'.

I asked Steve whether he could see anything and he said, "No", and I remember thinking, 'Thank God for that, he would probably have passed out'. He kept saying to me, "It's okay, it will be over in a minute"… and then the consultant lifted up this little thing all covered in blood and said, "You've got a lovely baby boy".

He was taken away immediately for tests and I'm not sure what they do, but he scored really highly and was pronounced fit and healthy. They gave him to Steve who gently laid him on my chest. We'd had lots of names in mind but suddenly I knew he had to be called Joseph. I suppose it was our way of thanking God that our baby was healthy when things had been so touch and go.

Maggie, 34, freelance marketing consultant, and Tony, 34, who runs his own marketing and promotional agency

"I can't do it, it's too painful"

"We can't time them, they're coming too quickly"

"I gripped Tony's shoulders and screamed, 'Something's coming'"

Tony and I had been trying for nearly two years to have our second child, and in some ways I'd almost forgotten about it. My periods were never regular and it wasn't until I was a good few weeks late that I decided to try a home pregnancy test. The positive result came as a bit of a shock. Instead of the rush of excitement and wild joy I'd experienced the first time round, I found myself almost complacent. I remember thinking, 'Oh, I'm pregnant again… hmm', and it suddenly dawned on me exactly what that meant. My first child, Jamie, was now four years old and at a stage where we no longer had to load up the car with pushchairs, carrycots and all the paraphernalia a baby needs. To be honest, the thought of having to go through all that again, along with months of sleepless nights, filled me with horror.

Although inwardly I loved the idea of being pregnant – the thought of a little baby growing inside me was a wonderful sensation – outwardly I really didn't revel in my stomach getting bigger and bigger, or my boobs expanding to Playmate of the Year proportions, and I couldn't wait to get the whole thing over with. As with Jamie, I was lucky and experienced no morning sickness, and basically sailed through the first six months. However, during the last stages I went through a very emotional state. I had waves of uncertainty about the new baby. At times I really wasn't sure that I wanted another child. In the main this was due to Jamie; I couldn't understand how I'd be able to love another child as much as I loved him. I didn't want to take anything away from Jamie, and the idea of another baby coming between us upset me greatly. At the same time I could see my independence disappearing, something I'd regained over the last couple of years, and I didn't relish giving it all up. The weeks passed and, although there were times when I felt

27

happy and looked forward to the birth, my fears still lurked constantly in the background.

My first labour had taken 22 hours and I'd only had the epidural two hours before Jamie was born. It was absolute hell, and Tony and I both decided this time it would be different. We planned to have only two children and so, as this was to be our last chance to experience childbirth, we wanted it to be as happy, relaxed and painfree as possible. The plan was to arrive at the hospital in plenty of time and be safely plugged up to the epidural before the contractions got really bad. On 31st May, the day the baby was officially due, I went into hospital for a scan because there was some worry the baby was too small. Luckily, the scan proved that everything was normal but just as I was about to leave, the doctor decided to, "just have a little feel up there". I remember saying to him afterwards, "That was a con", because it had been intensely painful. Looking back, I think he actually broke my cervix to hurry the whole thing along a bit. However, the general opinion was that the baby would be born within the week, and I was sent home to sit it out.

That night, at about 1am, I was woken up by a sort of wet sensation and my first thought was, 'Oh my gosh, I've wet the bed, how weird'. I remember thinking, as I got out of bed very sleepily, 'I'm a big girl now, I can't wet the bed at my age'. By the time I reached the bathroom I realised, with some relief, that my waters were breaking. I didn't panic at all, I just thought I'd better ring the hospital; they told me to make myself a cup of tea and come in fairly shortly.

Just then, I had the faintest imaginable sensation of contractions. I woke up Tony with the news, but he promptly fell back to sleep, and so I decided to have a shower. Halfway through washing my hair, I got the most agonising contraction – it was so bad I had to hang on to the showerhead for support. It was similar to pains I'd experienced in the final stages with Jamie, but at this point I really didn't expect another contraction for at least half an hour.

As I stepped out of the shower, another one hit me, probably three minutes after the last. I remember thinking, 'Wow, these are coming pretty fast', but I didn't panic as I still had hours and hours to go – or so I thought. By now, about 1.15, Tony had got himself together and called to me from the bedroom asking if I had any contractions yet and whether he should time them.

At that moment I got another one, and literally had to grab at pieces of furniture as I made my way back to the bedroom. I just looked at Tony and said, "We can't time them, they're coming too quickly, they're just waving over me". He realised how much pain I was in and then I think we both began to panic slightly. Tony practically carried me down the stairs and by 1.25 we were in the car.

It was the drive of Tony's life. The roads were clear and I don't think the speedometer dropped below 100mph. We jumped red lights, screeched around corners, and where normally I would have been scared out of my wits, I really couldn't care less. I just wanted to get there, I wanted him to go that fast. Anyway, I think we reached the hospital in five minutes, and it's normally at least a 15-minute journey. Later, Tony said he wished he'd been stopped by the police, because it was the one time he could legitimately prove why he was speeding!

As I got out of the car, I had a sensation of something dropping out of me; I literally had to put my hands between my legs to support myself. I don't know if the pain had clouded my judgement, or whether I'm just stupid, but at that moment I still didn't think I was about to have a baby. Quick labours to me took about four to five hours, so surely I still had plenty of time?

As the lift took us up to the labour ward, I was engulfed by a terrible, searing pain. I don't know how we made it to the nurses' station, but as we arrived I said, "Hello, my name is Maggie Appi, can I please have the epidural?" They showed us to the labour room and a midwife arrived. I begged for some pain relief but she very calmly said, "Yes, we'll organise that for you soon, Maggie, let's just get you on to the bed and see how far you're gone". Tony was trying to remain calm and they both helped me to undress, while I writhed around in agony. I think the midwife was thinking, 'Oh yes, I've seen this before, we'll get her on the bed and she'll only be 5cm dilated'.

As I climbed up I experienced the most horrendous contraction, I gripped Tony's shoulders and screamed, "Something's coming!" I can remember thinking, 'and I've still got my knickers on'. The midwife quickly examined me. "Yes, you're right, a baby's coming". She walked over to the door and called into the corridor, "Can I have some assistance please, a baby is about to be born".

I looked at her in horror. "What about the epidural, where's my epidural?" "I'm afraid it's too late for that Maggie, you're about to have your baby." My first thought was, 'I can't have this baby naturally, I'm not that brave!' But then two other midwives arrived and, with Tony by my side, they got me into position. One of them told me to start pushing and I suddenly realised the pain had stopped. I was still getting contractions because I had to push on them, but that intense, sweeping agony had subsided. I thought, 'Oh, this isn't too bad' and began to calm down. It was then that I realised I actually liked the idea of giving birth naturally – given the choice I still would have opted for the epidural – but that wasn't to be, and so I gritted my teeth and got on with it.

Pushing is very hard work and I quickly became exhausted with it. The pain was intensifying again and one of the midwives told me she could see the top of the baby's head. "One more push, Maggie, come on, one more," they all chorused. I began to push on the next contraction, but suddenly the pain was unbelievable; I thought, 'If I push harder, I'll rip apart'. I gripped Tony's arm, "I can't do it, it's too painful".

They were insisting I push, but instead I lay back and rested. It seemed to give me strength and I thought, 'Come on Mags, pull yourself together, let's get this baby born'. I prepared myself for the worst and pushed with all my might and strangely it wasn't as painful.

I think my body had expanded naturally and, within seconds, at 1.50am, after fifty minutes of labour, Daniel was born. He came out facing me, so I knew immediately he was a little boy. Just for a second, I was a little sad, because I knew I'd never have a girl, but I quickly got over it.

I didn't feel as emotional as I did with Jamie; when he was born Tony and I were crying and looking at him with absolute wonder. But I held Daniel and so did Tony; in fact Tony held him for longer than I did. Then we put him in his cot. I remember being quite happy for him to be there. They brought us tea and toast and Daniel was washed and weighed. Because of the time, Tony had to leave, and they gave Daniel to me to hold as we were wheeled down to the ward.

It was then that I fell in love with him. It hadn't been instant, as with Jamie, but the same magic was working, we were bonding and I knew without a shadow of a doubt that I could love them equally.

As for the sleepless nights and the baby paraphernalia, well... that's all part of the joy of being a parent, and I love every minute of it.

Viv, 29, supply teacher, and David, 32, professional hockey player

"I put on four stone, *four stone!*"

"I felt weak and trembly and thought, 'Hmm, I know this feeling'"

"I lay there eyeball to eyeball with this tiny new baby and thought, 'It's just you and me now'"

I didn't need a pregnancy test with my second baby, because the day before my period was due I felt very weak and trembly at my aerobics class and thought, 'Hmm, I know this feeling'. The baby was planned and David and I were absolutely delighted. As with my first baby, Elly, I felt sick every single day for the first three months. I never actually vomited, but all the same it was a pretty gruesome time. After that things went very well, but I began to put on quite a lot of weight. At 12 weeks I'd put on half a stone and I just kept getting bigger and bigger. It wasn't due to overeating, so I began to worry and pointed it out to the staff at the hospital each time I went for a check-up, but nothing was ever done about it. In the end I was around four stone overweight, *four stone!* You can't imagine how big I was. David came with me on my next hospital visit and gave them a bit of a hard time about it. Finally, the consultant was called. He checked my notes, reassured me that since my blood pressure was okay there really was nothing to worry about, and said that it was just one of those unfortunate side-effects of pregnancy. On top of this I developed the most awful heartburn, which I just couldn't get rid of, and towards the end I became slightly depressed and weepy.

I'd been told quite early on that the baby was breech, but this is very common and they normally turn of their own accord. However, at 35 weeks the baby was still in the same position, and I was sent to have an X-ray to measure my pelvis and also to have the baby weighed. It was nearly 7lbs and I still had over a month to go!

They told me that the baby was unlikely to turn now and that because I'd had to have a forceps delivery with Elly, there would be no way I'd be able to push this baby out myself. So we all agreed that a Caesarean would be the safest option for us both.

A date was set and then they said that if my waters broke or I went into labour by myself, we should call for an ambulance immediately so that I could lie down on the way in. This struck me as rather alarmist and I suggested that since I surely wouldn't have the baby within ten minutes I could go by car, but they were adamant, so I agreed. Anyway my waters hadn't broken with Elly, so I really didn't think they would this time either.

Luckily, David's on BUPA, and with this you get a single room and the consultant to deliver you, so we made an appointment to see him on 30th December, three weeks before the baby was due.

Over Christmas I was very hormonal and weepy and my enormous size really got me down. We'd seen mainly family over the holidays and with the impending arrival of the new baby we realised we'd be out of action socially for quite a while, so on the spur of the moment we decided to throw a small party. People started arriving around sixish and by 7 o'clock there were between 15 to 20 people here.

I was really enjoying myself and talking to a friend of mine who'd had twins. She was holding one and then I noticed her husband had put down the other one so he could drink his beer. Typical! I scooped him up and carried on chatting, when suddenly I felt this hot liquid running down my legs. I knew immediately that my waters had broken and so I said, "Excuse me", and headed for the downstairs loo, still clutching the baby.

By this time I was absolutely awash, it seemed liked gallons of water were pouring out of me. You hear about these women who break in Sainsbury's and it must be just so embarrassing for them. Anyway, I slammed the bathroom door, looked at this baby I was still holding, and wailed, "What do I do now?"

I didn't know whether to stand up, sit on the loo, or lie down – you know, because they'd put it into my head about lying down. So there I am standing up, sitting down, with this baby still in my arms and I said to myself, 'Okay, get a grip'.

I thought I should at least let David know, and opened the bathroom door only to hear him yelling at the top of his voice, "Oh God, whose spilt their beer all over the carpet?" I was mortified, as can you imagine, and quickly shut the bathroom door again. Eventually, the girl I'd been talking to, who was left wondering why I'd run off like that, and what this stuff was all over the floor, came and tapped on the door.

"Are you okay in there Viv?" "No, I'm not." I let her in and gratefully handed over the baby, then fled upstairs to change into some leggings. I was running around the bedroom throwing God knows what into a bag, stopping every now and then to lie down, getting up, throwing more bits into the bag and was basically in a complete frenzy. Meanwhile, downstairs, David had been told what was happening and was in a bit of a frenzy himself. He had already phoned for an ambulance and then realised he had to phone the consultant, whom we hadn't even met yet, and he didn't have his number. Apparently he was telling everyone not to panic, while running in and out of the room saying, "Who do I phone?" It was only when a friend, who'd had three kids, said, "Look David, stand still, calm down, where are Viv's notes? All the numbers will be on there".

By this time all the world and his dog had been in to see how I was doing and it was only as an afterthought that David came in to see me himself! He rushed off again and then I heard him shouting, "Viv, Viv, the ambulance is here, quick, quick". I remember literally running down the stairs saying, "I'm here, I'm here" only to be confronted by the ambulance man saying, "Steady on luv, no need to rush is there?" I realised what I must have looked like and tried to regain my composure, "No, no, of course not, you're quite right".

We left the party with people shouting their encouragement and then I heard David say, "Carry on drinking lads, I'll be back in a few hours". The ambulance pulled away and the driver shouted back to me, "Normally it's the custom for the father to follow the ambulance" as David sped by in his car…

After a few minutes I realised I'd left without saying goodbye to Elly. It would have been the last time I'd see her as my only child and I felt so guilty, like I'd just ditched her. I remember getting quite lip-trembly and feeling really sad that we hadn't had those last moments together, just the two of us. Although my waters had broken, I still wasn't having any contractions and I didn't feel that I was in labour at all. I lay there thinking, 'Um, well you're going to have a baby today'. I felt almost detached from it, I suppose it was because I wasn't in any pain. We arrived at the hospital and there was David, looking calm and collected, with a cup of tea in his hands. We had to get ready for theatre and that was quite fun because David had to get togged up in the green outfit with the hat, mask and everything. I wasn't hurting at all and it was like going on an adventure together. David keep doing these *M.A.S.H.* impressions and we were having a really good giggle. They wheeled us into another room and there was a line you weren't allowed to cross unless your shoes had been covered. I think David got a bit jittery at this point. I had opted for the epidural so I could stay awake throughout the birth and, since I'd had one with Elly, I knew what to expect and wasn't frightened at all. I felt very in control of the situation and thought, 'This is going to be really good'.

At that moment I began to get contractions so I was given the epidural fairly quickly. I remember lying on the operating table and the anaesthetist pinching my stomach really hard to see if I could still feel anything. When I was completely numb, the consultant explained to me that I would be able to feel sensations in my stomach, perhaps a bit of pulling around and the incision being made, but absolutely no pain. I didn't feel at all frightened and was really enjoying myself until they put the screen over me, which seemed to be right up against my face, and suddenly I felt totally closed in and out of control. My hands were down by my side and I wanted to hold on to David, but was so scared of moving them that I asked if it would be okay. They looked at me as if I was some kind of loon and said, "Yes, of course you can".

After that I began to feel things happening and I even felt them making the incision and it's true, you really can't feel any pain at all. However, after a while I did begin to feel a slight pain and could definitely feel my contractions; I remember hearing my voice like a tiny little child saying to all these important people, "Excuse me, I can feel contractions". I asked if it was because I was scared and they said, "Oh yes, yes", and it made me think it was just my mind playing tricks. But afterwards David said they were making signs saying, 'Wop up the epidural'.

At this point it all stopped for a little while and then they gave me some sedation because I'd obviously shown signs of being a bit of a wobbler. That made me a bit away with the fairies and after that I wasn't quite aware of what was happening.

The next thing I remember is someone saying, "Right, we're going to lift the baby out now", and again they explained I would feel it but it wouldn't hurt, which was true. It was like someone massaging my tummy and a loud sort of sucking sound as they pulled my baby out. I heard them say, "Yes, well you can tell by the bottom bits it's a girl" and I thought, 'What an ungainly way of putting it', and then seemed to slip back into oblivion.

Poor David was really frightened at this point because all he could see was his new daughter being rugby tackled across the room to be cleaned up and me looking like I was dead. We realised later on that they always whisk breech babies away quickly because they come out feet first and as a result get a lot of fluid in their mouths.

As this was all going on around me I suddenly started to shake uncontrollably, I was literally bouncing around and I began to cry because I just couldn't stop it. They explained that it was a mixture of the sedation and epidural and just me throwing a bit of a wobbler. They gave me some more sedation and then I vaguely remember David holding the baby while they stitched me up.

David went home to see Elly and I was sent to the recovery room with the baby. Even though I was so out of it I remember lying there almost eyeball to eyeball with this tiny new baby and thinking, 'Hmm... it's just you and me now'. A midwife came in and tried to persuade me to feed her and, although every instinct told me this was the right thing to do, I just couldn't get my body together.

The first time I had the epidural I had no problems at all, it wore off and everything was fine, but this time I was lying there talking to the midwife and all of a sudden I saw something jump at the end of the bed. I thought it was a small animal. I remember saying, "My God, there's something in the bed, what the hell is it?" The midwife laughingly explained that it was my feet. I couldn't feel them but I could see them. My feet were kicking up and down and I really tried to control them but I couldn't – it was bizarre.

For the rest of the night I was still quite influenced by the sedation and it wasn't until the next day, when everything had worn off, that I felt we really bonded. Libby was so beautiful, I just couldn't stop looking at her. You know, no matter what your experience is, it's always worth it in the end.

Melinda, 42, career in public relations with her own successful company

"For some inane reason everyone thinks you're gaa-gaa"

"My conclusion is, you just want what you get"

"Oh my God, nobody mentioned forceps"

Three months to become pregnant! Wow, I was over the moon, absolutely elated. In fact, I was almost too scared to do the second test in case it didn't come up purple again. Although I had been thinking about having a baby for some years, the timing was never just right, mainly because of social circumstances and a very hectic working schedule. I suppose the catalyst, the precipitating thing, was that, at 38, I simply fell desperately in love and could think of no greater expression of that love than to conceive his child.

As my pregnancy progressed I went to great lengths to disguise it at work. I've seen too many female colleagues with their credibility shot to pieces once the big news was announced. For some inane reason, everyone thinks you're gaa-gaa and that all your decisions are emotionally-based rather than rational.

Also, because of my age, I was offered the option of having an amniocentesis, which tests for Down's syndrome, and this can sometimes result in spontaneous abortion. So I didn't want to tell everyone in case I ended up being one of the unlucky ones. The Bart's Test, so called because it is performed at St Bartholomew's hospital in London, is a combination scan and blood test which gives the statistical likelihood of having a Down's syndrome child. I think mine was a one in 849 chance.

At five months I had breakthrough bleeding. It was only a little spotting, but it absolutely terrified me. I grabbed everything I could read on the subject and rang everyone I knew who'd ever been pregnant. The general opinion was that there was nothing to worry about and a scan proved that they were right, but the whole episode was a real nightmare. I just kept thinking, 'Please God, don't let me lose this baby'. In general, though, I was deliriously happy. I glowed with health – you know the glow people associate with pregnant women – and emotionally I felt at one with the world.

At six months I realised that my relationship with the father of my child was not as stable as I had imagined. Very sadly, we parted, and I found myself a single mother. Luckily, I am financially secure in my own right but, as you can imagine, I underwent a lot of violent emotional feelings about the whole situation. Nevertheless, I was so thrilled about being pregnant and so desperate to keep the baby, that I very quickly got things into perspective and back on an even keel.

At this stage, I had already decided to have the baby privately and made a point of seeing a number of obstetricians until I found one I could relate to. It was very important to me to have somebody who would understand my situation and be kind and sympathetic. One chap I came across actually said he couldn't guarantee that he would deliver me personally, as he might be at a dinner party or away shooting!

In the end I rang a doctor friend who recommended an obstetrician at the Portland Hospital in London. We met and I clicked with him immediately; I knew I wasn't going to be treated like another faceless person. He explained to me that he nearly always induces his ladies so that he can deliver the babies personally, and between us we decided upon 3rd November.

At 32 weeks I went in for a final scan and asked the sex of my baby. When they said it was a boy I was ecstatic, which seemed funny at the time because all along I'd been hoping for a girl. My conclusion is that you just want what you get.

On the morning of 2nd November I woke up feeling really excited. I would be going into hospital that evening. It was a strange day, my bag was packed, everything was ready and, although I had a lot of last minute things to do to keep me busy, the time seemed to drag.

Finally, it was time to go and I arrived at the hospital around 6pm. The plan was that at midnight I would be given a pessary and then another one in the morning, which would soften my cervix and induce my labour.

I went to bed just after midnight but was woken at three in the morning by quite strong contractions, which really frightened me. This wasn't supposed to happen! I rang for the midwife who duly arrived and confirmed I was in labour. I began to panic. My obstetrician was still at home in bed and the anaesthetist who was booked to give me an epidural didn't come on duty until 8am.

They moved me to the labour ward and rang for the night duty doctor. By this time I was beginning to climb the walls with the pain. I could hear other women screaming and I now realised why; all I could think was, 'Where is the epidural?' I was so sure I'd made the right decision to have one, because at that point I'd really had enough. Different midwives came and went, but there wasn't any one person just to hold my hand or encourage me. In those few hours I couldn't have felt more alone.

They finally organised the epidural at 6am, when I was 3cms dilated, and the relief from the pain flooded through me. The difference half an hour later was remarkable. I was sitting up, on the phone to friends and colleagues, watching a news item about a project I was heavily involved in, and all thoughts about the fairly imminent arrival of my child seemed to have slipped into the background. I was still happily in this frame of mind when the obstetrician arrived, examined me, and said that my baby would be born within the next half an hour.

During the following 20 minutes I had great waves of emotion that racked my body. I would burst into tears and sob away, then it would stop and then it would start again. There was lots of activity going on around me: midwives were checking my contractions; and I suddenly realised that my obstetrician was all scrubbed up and in full green theatre outfit, looking as though he was about to perform a major operation instead of just deliver a baby. I was quite shocked by the sight of this, but he reassured me that everything was fine and it was now time to start pushing.

The midwife monitored my contractions and indicated when I should bear down. I was surprised to hear that after only three attempts the baby's head was crowning. I realised that I must have been having very strong contractions for things to be this far advanced, but of course with the epidural you just don't feel anything. Then the obstetrician suddenly produced a pair of forceps and I thought, 'Oh my God, nobody mentioned forceps'.

He explained that the baby's shoulder was stuck and the forceps would make his birth that much easier. I had to have an episiotomy and, you know, when you're pregnant, thinking about these things which always seem to involve knives or needles really terrifies you. Yet it was over in a flash and I wasn't even aware that it had been done. My legs were put into stirrups, which is the most ungainly position, and I saw the doctor get to work with the forceps. I couldn't actually see what he was doing, but I could see a sheet of blood right down the front of his gown. Although I seemed to be detached from it, because of the lack of pain, it was still pretty disconcerting. Within seconds, he pulled a baby from between my legs and plonked him on to my chest... my son was born.

At first I couldn't quite believe that this was my baby. In some ways I didn't really feel as though I had been that involved in his birth. Of course I had, I'd given birth – but it had all been so controlled. I didn't bond with my baby immediately, I suppose because he had been real to me from the moment I discovered he was a boy at 32 weeks. To be honest, I was more concerned about my current business deal. You have to understand that I'd been in business for more than 20 years and that was my life.

For the next two days it was business as usual... and then my milk came in. From that moment on my world turned upside down. Here was this tiny baby who depended entirely on me; I was completely absorbed by him; he became the focus of my life. I couldn't have cared less if the Prime Minister had been on the phone... I had become a Mother!

Judy, 31, part-time language teacher, and John, 34, overseas property developer

"From the moment I knew the sex of my baby I felt I knew him"

"I seemed to have wires coming out of me everywhere"

"I'd rather have pain relief and try to enjoy the birth"

I'd recently had a miscarriage so I was pleased to be pregnant again, although obviously I didn't feel as relaxed as I might have done. I had been 11 weeks when I'd miscarried so I was very apprehensive indeed. In the second month I had a loss of blood, and was petrified that the same thing was going to happen again. I was put on instant bed rest and by the third month the doctors were satisfied that the danger had passed and the baby was fine. I did begin to relax more, but not entirely. Consequently, I didn't really enjoy my pregnancy.

I was in Italy for the first seven months because my husband was on an assignment out there and, fortunately, our circumstances were such that I was able to join him. I had all the normal checks and a follow-up scan at five months and on that occasion discovered that the baby was a boy. At that stage in my pregnancy I wanted to know as much as possible, so when the doctor asked me if I wanted to know the sex of the baby, I jumped at the chance.

From that moment on I felt I knew him. I could imagine what he would be like and it made the pregnancy very secure, which was great after all the problems I'd had. Although my husband's contract in Italy still had a few months to run, I returned home to spend Christmas with my parents. I was getting big and cumbersome and felt that I needed to be home. I went to my local hospital to discuss the birth and told them that I very much wanted to wait and see what happened and not make any definite plans, as I didn't know what to expect or how my labour would progress.

In my last month my blood pressure shot up and I was diagnosed as having pre-eclampsia. The dreadful thing about this condition is that your body really swells up, and I looked awful. The medical profession really don't know very much about it, what the causes are, or how to treat it. It sends your blood pressure sky high and the only thing that eases the situation is to get as much bed rest as possible. The swelling wasn't painful or even uncomfortable in itself, but it can be life threatening for the baby and mother, so I was very worried.

I spent the remaining four weeks of my pregnancy in and out of hospital; they only allowed me home when my blood pressure dropped, and I literally wasn't allowed to do anything. I'd been told that if my blood pressure didn't stabilise I would have to have an emergency Caesarean.

They checked my blood pressure every four hours and it was a real strain because I knew that if it went any higher they would whisk me down to the operating theatre. In the middle of this my husband returned home and I was hoping that his arrival would ease the strain I was under and perhaps in turn help to lower my blood pressure. Fat chance!

At 39 weeks things still hadn't improved and, although I wasn't in an emergency situation, the doctors decided to induce me. So I was told, "Today is the day" and was taken down to the delivery suite. I was really excited. After all the ups and downs, something positive was finally going to happen. I was given three pessaries, which I found quite painful, and John and I settled down to wait for the big event. This was in the morning and by mid-day we were still waiting. Tea-time came and went and by the end of the day absolutely nothing had happened, not even the slightest twinge. So, with great disappointment, I was sent back to the antenatal ward.

The next day I went down again, was given more pessaries and still nothing happened. Eventually the doctors said that they would leave me over the weekend, which I was really pleased about, because not only was I very sore by now, but two days in the delivery suite and no baby was quite soul-destroying.

On the Sunday they allowed me home for lunch, and as John was driving me back to the hospital, I began to feel this dull ache in my back and I thought, 'I wonder if this is it'. I didn't say anything to anybody, and it didn't get worse, so I went to bed that night not really thinking too much about it.

At 6.30am I woke up with fairly strong contractions but, after all I'd been through, I still couldn't believe things were really moving at last. I called the nurse and asked if she could put me on the foetal heart monitor, so that we could see whether the contractions were registering or not. It was confirmed that I was in the early stages of labour, and then it was just a case of waiting.

I'd been told by the consultants that it would be sensible for me to have an epidural because it helps to lower your blood pressure. I think the idea is that because you feel no pain you don't get so wound up and therefore your blood pressure drops. At this point I felt quite relaxed, I knew the delivery suite and I knew the nurses, so I had a fairly clear picture in my head of how things were going to be.

I had breakfast and then took a long leisurely bath. I think I must have been in there for an hour or more. At about mid-morning my husband arrived, and together we timed the contractions. They were coming every five minutes but were bearable and I was coping with them quite easily. I went down to the hospital shop to buy some barley sugar because someone had told me it was a good thing to have when you're in labour.

I had just collected my change when I was overcome by the severity of a contraction. I clutched the side of the counter and waited for it to pass. It was a really intense pain in my stomach. My husband helped me back to the ward and I suddenly realised I was incredibly hungry. Thankfully, it was lunchtime and I devoured my food like a woman possessed; it was almost like an instinct within me to eat as much as I could and build up my strength. I even ate the leftovers from the girl next to me.

Over the next few hours my contractions got steadily worse and worse. I wanted to see a doctor but none was available. I got quite weepy, all I wanted to do was find out what was happening. I went up to one of the nurses' stations and promptly burst into tears. The pain was causing me to double up over the table. They were coming every five minutes and each one lasted 40 to 45 seconds. The nurses apologised for leaving me so long; apparently there had been an emergency situation – a lady had arrived at only 26 weeks pregnant so it had been all hands on deck.

They took me up to the delivery suite and I was told that I was 4cms dilated. The midwife congratulated me for doing so much work on my own, although it wasn't really by choice! I actually felt quite deflated because I was hoping it would be time to start pushing. At this stage I felt I was ready for the epidural and while they went to summon up the anaesthetist the midwife gave me a shot of Pethidine. The sensation was really wonderful, I felt like I was floating on air and I almost fell asleep. When the anaesthetist arrived I got quite annoyed at having to be disturbed because it was the first time in ten hours that I'd actually been comfortable.

The epidural was brilliant because suddenly the pain was gone and it wasn't like being in labour at all. Obviously, everything was going on, but I wasn't aware of it. I remember thinking, 'Oh my God, some women are paralysed', but once they'd done it, it was such a relief I didn't care. I never really planned on having a totally natural labour. Although you don't really know what the pain is going to be like, I wasn't prepared to be a martyr. I'd rather have pain relief and try to enjoy the birth.

After that it was just hours and hours of labour. I seemed to have wires coming out of me everywhere. Because of the pre-eclampsia I had to have a blood pressure cuff on the whole time which would swell up every five minutes and give a reading. I had drips on both arms, the foetal heart monitor and the epidural. After a while it began to wear off and I started to get some movement back in my legs. I was feeling really fidgety and hemmed in and, much to the annoyance of the staff, I kept trying to move around. So I guess it was my own fault that the epidural partly came out and therefore wasn't working as well as it should have been.

The pain came back with a vengeance, it was unbearable; I literally went from nothing to second stage labour contractions. While I waited for the anaesthetist to come back, they gave me some gas and air to help calm things down a bit. The contractions were coming every two to three minutes and I found it really difficult to cope. I remember at one point being abusive to the doctors and midwives. John was great, poor man, all I did was bark instructions at him: "gas, flannel, water, hand". But he never lost his temper, just gently tried to keep me calm the whole time.

The epidural was eventually sorted out and I experienced that great sense of relief again. Things went on fairly smoothly for another hour or so and then about 8pm it was suggested that my waters were broken to hurry things along a bit. I remember being quite surprised at all this murky water coming out and one of the nurses told me that meconium was present, which might indicate that the baby was in distress. They didn't seem too worried about it, but said that things would have to proceed fairly quickly.

Because they weren't worried I wasn't worried either – everybody seemed to know what they were doing, so I just let them get on with it. It wasn't long after that, I guess about 9.30, that they said I'd fully dilated and could start pushing. It was awful because I just couldn't get my act together at all. They kept saying, "Push, push" and nothing was happening. I just felt I wasn't doing it properly. They tried to encourage me by saying the baby would be born before 11 and I remember looking constantly at the time thinking, 'I can't do this, why can't I do this?'

By 11.30 it was all getting too much for me and I asked how much longer it was going to take. The baby's heartbeat was fine and I was urged to carry on. I tried as hard as I could but by 1.30am I was literally begging them to help me in some way to deliver the baby. I just didn't feel that I could do it on my own, I was so tired, I couldn't bear it any longer. The time passed by and eventually I gave up – I was pushing but it was so half-hearted, mainly because I didn't have any strength left.

At 3am a doctor came in and said they would probably have to do a Caesarean because the head hadn't even crowned. I was so relieved when he said this because all I wanted was for the baby to be born. I was asked if I wanted to have the baby using the epidural or by general anaesthetic. In my mind, at that time, there was no doubt about it. I just didn't want to participate any more at all and asked for the general anaesthetic.

Suddenly everything seemed to turn into an emergency; doctors appeared from everywhere and within seconds I was being wheeled down to the operating theatre. John had to stay outside and I remember, as they closed the doors, noticing how forlorn he looked. My legs were put into stirrups and my pubic area was shaved. I just lay there with my eyes shut, totally still. One of the nurses joked that I looked as if I'd already been knocked out.

Two doctors arrived fully kitted out in their green gowns and masks and said, "How about one last push before we get on with it?" So I gave one last push and then they said, "Give another push", and I was so annoyed. Why did they say one last push if they didn't mean it. I suddenly became aware that they were all laughing, literally falling about.

The senior surgeon pulled his mask off and said, "My dear, you've had a lucky escape, your baby's head is out". Well, I just couldn't believe it, I was totally miffed. I'd put no effort whatsoever into those last two pushes and thought it was all a complete waste of time. I gave one final push and then these little feet landed on me and they told me it was a boy. I smiled and said, "I know", to which they looked a bit puzzled and went off to fetch John.

He was obviously still under the impression that I'd had the baby by Caesarean and nearly fell over when he walked in to see me waving at him and wide awake. We were both so stunned by the turn of events that it wasn't until we got back to the delivery suite that it began to sink in.

I remember that moment vividly. It was snowing heavily outside and the wind was howling against the windows. The hospital was very quiet because it was still early in the morning and the three of us lay on the bed, snuggling together. My labour had been long and at times indescribably painful but, to this day, whenever I see snow, I get a lovely warm feeling inside.

Ros, 28, City broker, and Gavin, 32, architect

"I used to find myself falling asleep at dinner parties"

"They asked me if I wanted any pain relief and I said, 'Yes, yes. Definitely'"

"It was the best and most exciting thing that's ever happened to me"

Gavin and I decided we wanted to have children and, amazingly, I fell pregnant the following month, so we were very happy. The first few months were awful. I was tired, really, really tired. So much so, that I used to find myself falling asleep at dinner parties – until somebody would wake me because I was about to fall into my soup or something.

I set my sights on 12 weeks, having been told that it would probably all be over by then, but it was more like 16 weeks and it actually got worse. Eventually it did stop and everyone kept saying how well I looked. I didn't put on any extra weight and the rest of the pregnancy was really easy. I worked up until three weeks before the baby was due and found it very strenuous; work was the last place I wanted to be by that time.

We really wanted to keep an open mind about how we were going to have the baby, but I did decide that I would try to avoid an epidural as much as possible. I hate needles and the thought of someone sticking a needle and tube in my back was terrifying. However, realistically, I knew that if things got really bad I'd certainly go for it.

I wanted to discover as much as possible about what giving birth was really like. I didn't come across many books that told it as it really was and in the end, I guess like everybody else, I resorted to asking friends and relatives. Some would say, "It's like having appendicitis", and others were quick to reassure me that it wasn't too bad, it was manageable. So there wasn't much else I could do but to wait and see for myself.

Quite late into the pregnancy my Mother gave me a book by an American called Dick Read, and although it had been written in the

Fifties and was a bit old-fashioned, it was really interesting. It explained how, for the first time, relaxation techniques were replacing heavy sedation to help women cope with the pain of labour. I was already practising relaxation and breathing through my antenatal classes and so I found it very useful.

A couple of days before my due date, I woke up at about 6.30 in the morning feeling distinctly odd; I can't describe it, other than feeling that something was 'happening'. I didn't think it could be the beginning of my labour because I didn't feel any particular pains; I was just a bit unsettled and couldn't go back to sleep. It didn't unnerve me though and I just sort of went along with it.

I got up to go to the toilet and was fairly convinced that I'd had a show. I woke up Gavin and said, "Look, I think I might be in labour". There wasn't anything definite other than the show, I just had a strange inner feeling. I rang the hospital and told the midwife exactly what had happened, but she said that it didn't really mean anything: "Your baby could be born today or next week, see how you get on and give us a ring if you start to get contractions".

I put down the phone down and thought, 'Okay then, fine, things are probably going to move quite slowly'. We were both pretty relaxed until about 9 o'clock, when I had my first contraction. Then I had another one at ten past, and another at 20 past, and so on. I said, "They're coming every five minutes, didn't the hospital say that when they're coming this quickly we should go in?" Gavin joked, "No, no. It says in this Dick Read book of yours that in the first stages of labour women can do light housework, so get on with the washing up!" I did say it was written in the Fifties!

I went up to get my things together, leaving Gavin downstairs in the hope that he would organise everything. The contractions were coming thick and fast and I could hear Gavin faffing around. I called to him, "Come up here, I can't cope with this". He still didn't materialise, so I screamed at him, "Gavin, what are you doing? We've got to go". I found him in the kitchen frantically trying to smash up ice-cubes and squeeze them into the thermos flask. He was obviously still under the impression that this was going to take a long time – but I knew differently, because minute by minute the contractions were getting closer and closer.

Gavin rang for a taxi and I could hear him waffling on with no sense of urgency. I said, "Don't bother with the taxi, call my sister". Luckily, she lives just across the road and I knew she could be here almost immediately. But she had different ideas and told Gavin that she'd be over in about 15 minutes, as she had to put her makeup on. I grabbed the phone and said, "Get over here *now!*" Two minutes later we were getting into the car. It was around 9.50 by now and the contractions were coming every minute. I could barely walk.

When we arrived at the hospital they really didn't take me very seriously. I'm sure they just thought, 'Oh no, another panicky first-time mother'. A midwife arrived and asked me for a sample and I said, "There's absolutely no way anything's coming out except the baby". She stuck me in the bathroom anyway and asked me to try, and I remember sitting on the floor, because I couldn't stand, until they came to collect me. I was in the middle of a contraction and the midwife said, "That was a very long one, how often are they coming?" As I began to answer another one came and I was quickly put into the delivery room.

All of a sudden people just descended upon me and I could see them opening up bags and trying to pull on gloves and hats. They asked me if I wanted any pain relief and I said, "Yes, yes. Definitely". They gave me the gas and air but took it away again after five minutes – apparently you relax so much that you don't push, and I had already gone into the third stage of labour. I remember they had to peel my hand off the mask; it was a really powerful feeling, like I was floating on the ceiling.

I completely retreated from the world, I could hear people talking but it seemed so far away. I can remember pushing and pushing for ages, it was really hard work – I felt like I was running in a marathon. I was really scared about having an episiotomy and I'd read somewhere that if you smile when the baby's being born, it relaxes your muscles and you're less likely to tear. So I was trying to concentrate on smiling and making every effort to relax and, although it was quite painful, I certainly found it helped.

I was quite shocked at how quickly my little girl was born. She arrived at 11.30 in the morning and Gavin and I were ecstatic. It was the best and most exciting thing that's ever happened to me. It's so funny because you have this thing growing inside you and you know it's there because it kicks you and you get to know it, but it feels completely different when this little person is actually born.

I couldn't quite believe that one minute she'd been inside me and the next she wasn't, it's all quite mind-boggling. We were both in tears and so happy. It's not the kind of happiness you could ever feel normally… To experience it, I guess you've just got to have a baby.

Mai-Britt, 31, air stewardess, and Paul, 41, who runs his own plumbing business

"I could see on their faces that they thought, 'Oh dear, it's too late, it's gone'"

"It's upside down, the little devil"

"Oh no, not again… and then the bleeding started"

Paul and I were away skiing at the time and I thought I'd caught a chill because I had to keep stopping every five minutes to do a wee. Very annoying, especially when you've got half a dozen zips to contend with and four different layers of clothing. Anyway the 'chill' continued when we got home and after a couple of weeks I started to get funny little pains in my stomach, so I decided to go to the doctor's because it just wasn't clearing up.

My period was late and I did a urine test before I went because I knew the doctor would only assume that I was pregnant, which of course I wasn't. I did the test in the morning, and it was positive. I couldn't believe it, I'd paid out £10 for the bloody thing and it didn't even work.

Paul said, "Well maybe it's right, perhaps you are pregnant". I just laughed, "No, no, how can I be, we haven't done anything to get pregnant. It must be something to do with that chill I caught skiing".

I explained my symptoms to my GP and said that I'd done a pregnancy test that hadn't worked and could she please tell me what was wrong. Her reaction was to laugh, she just sat there laughing at me, and said, "Well, it sounds to me as if you are pregnant". I said, "Look you're not taking me seriously, we've been using contraception, it's not possible, whatever it is I know I caught it on holiday". She laughed even more and said, "Okay, let's have a look". Ten minutes later I walked out of the surgery in a daze. Wow, I was pregnant.

I think every emotion possible hit me on the way back to the car. I was excited but frightened, how could this have happened without my knowing? It was as if I had been betrayed by my body and, anyway, I

51

wasn't even sure this was the right time to have a baby. For Paul, it was the best news he'd ever had, but he didn't pressurise me and said no matter what he thought the final decision was mine.

I thought long and hard about it and realised there never is a right time to have a baby. You can't just say, 'Well, I'll get another one of you next year, when you fit into my personal planner more easily'. Once I'd made the decision I just felt elated. 'Yes, we're going to have a little baby and that's good, really good.'

At first I felt wonderful, really healthy, and then at about eight weeks I had a particularly bad bout of flu. I was getting over the worst of it and was on the phone to my Mother when I felt a really warm rush between my legs. I thought, 'Hell, what on earth is this', and then I saw fresh red blood. I literally screamed my head off, which must have been awful for my mother, at home in Denmark, because all she could hear was her daughter wailing, "Oh my God, no, please, please".

I flung down the phone, ran to the toilet and there was even more blood. I was on my knees praying to God or whoever, "Don't do this to me, don't take my child away", but it kept on coming and then I started to pass what looked like lumps of liver. I was too frightened to stand up, I was afraid that if I did my baby would fall out. The phone rang again in the kitchen, I thought it was my Mother but in fact it was my friend Nina. "Nina, Nina, listen, I'm bleeding. What shall I do?" I was shaking and crying and she said, "Hold on, I'll come straight round and take you to your doctor".

I was rushed straight into the surgery expecting the worst but my GP said, "Your cervix is closed, which is a very, very good sign, but you are bleeding quite heavily. To be on the safe side we're going to have to scan you".

The hospital couldn't fit me in there and then so we had to wait until the following day. I was quite convinced that something very bad had happened. At eight weeks the baby is only 2-3cms long and after seeing those lumps I was sure I'd miscarried.

As they ran the scanner over my stomach I prepared myself for the worst and then suddenly, there it was, a little creature with two arms, two legs and, yes, a heartbeat. "Oh my God, look, our baby is okay." We were both crying with relief and happiness. The hospital doctor assured me that everything was fine, the lining of the womb was intact and other than, "It's just one of those things", they had no real explanation for what had happened.

I was still bleeding quite heavily and deep inside I felt really worried; it seemed so weird, surely this wasn't normal? Yet there had been a perfectly healthy-looking foetus up on the screen, and so I just tried to accept that everything was okay and put it out of my mind as best I could.

The next day was Saturday and Paul and I decided to go for a walk. We couldn't take our eyes off all these babies and parents. What are they like, parents? This weird society that we were soon going to be a part of? They seemed to be like some kind of secret clan and we wondered what we would be like when our turn came. We were having so much fun, we were on cloud nine all weekend, we were going to have a baby and it just filled us both with so much happiness. On Monday morning Paul went off to work, and I was just coming down the stairs with a cup of tea when, without any kind of warning, I had a contraction. It was heavy and painful and I knew instantly what it was. I just went pale, 'No, no, not again'… And then the bleeding started. I rang Paul to come home straight away and phoned for an ambulance. It was so sad, after our lovely weekend when we were sure everything was fine – it was so unfair I just couldn't believe it.

At the hospital they confirmed that I was having contractions and asked if I wanted any pain relief. I said, "Yes", but as they came at me with the needle I said, "No, no, I don't want it, take it away". I was definitely in pain but something inside me said, 'Don't do it'. I could see on their faces that they thought, 'Oh dear, it's too late, it's gone'. The doctor said that my cervix had opened and that he would give me a D&C just to remove any stray bits and that within three months I'd be able to try for another baby.

I was crying, Paul was crying, we'd really wanted this baby and now it was all over. They sent me off for a scan and of course the technician didn't know what was going on, to him I was just another pregnant lady. So when he said, "There's your lovely little baby", I just went into shock. What was going on?

At first I thought there was somebody else's baby up on the screen… and then it began to sink in. There it was again, this perfectly formed little baby waving at us. The doctor was called in and he was as amazed as we were. Nobody could work it out. I had all the symptoms of an early miscarriage and yet there was no doubt that I was still pregnant.

I stayed in hospital so that they could keep an eye on me. Every morning I dreaded looking at the press-on towel which, without fail, was full of blood. But I didn't have any more pain, and after four days they sent me home and told me to rest in bed. Resting wouldn't guarantee that I wouldn't miscarry, but at least I wouldn't feel guilty if things did go wrong. I stayed in bed for two weeks. I kept getting pain and the bleeding still hadn't stopped.

In the end I couldn't stand it and went to see my GP who said, "These symptoms are all perfectly normal after a miscarriage". I nearly fell off my chair. "What do you mean, a miscarriage." She then went on to explain that the hospital notes after my first scan had shown a collapsed sac and another perfectly normal sac with a foetus inside – which meant that I had in fact been carrying twins and had lost one baby. I don't know why the scanning person hadn't told me the truth, it would have saved me weeks of agony and distress. Because the notes from the first scan had been sent back to my GP on the Friday, this meant that when I was taken into hospital on the Monday the doctors on duty understandably had no idea what had happened. Of course I was relieved finally to find out the truth, now it all made sense: the bleeding was due to the scarring from the miscarried twin. But, I felt cheated and angry, it didn't seem to be anybody's fault, yet I didn't believe how something like that could have happened.

Everyone tried to reassure me that I would maintain the existing pregnancy but it didn't stop me worrying. The worst thing was the fresh blood every morning – because my body was maintaining a healthy baby, it took ages to heal the scar from the other one. In the end I didn't stop bleeding until about five months, by which time I felt I ought to have had shares in Boots for all the press-on towels I'd bought.

When I finally got round to thinking about how I wanted to have the baby it was quite late on in my pregnancy. At first I wanted to go home to Denmark, mainly because of the language barrier. I speak fluent English, but nevertheless when you are frightened or in pain you'd rather hear somebody reassuring you in your native tongue. You know, 'push, push' wouldn't mean as much to me as 'skub, skub' in Danish.

We talked about renting a flat there and Paul commuting backwards and forwards. Because I'm an air stewardess the cost wouldn't be a problem. So at six months I flew home. But I missed Paul so much, each time the baby kicked I wanted to tell him and it just wasn't the same telling my Mother. I realised very quickly that it was wrong, I had made my home in England and that's where we should be.

The next idea was to have the baby at home, but my doctor advised me otherwise. She felt that, as it was a first baby, and considering the complications I'd already had, the risks were too high. At the end of the day, we opted for the local hospital. They had a lovely birthing room with nice furnishings, all very homely and comfortable, and I felt at ease with the idea of having my baby there.

At 36 weeks I had a hospital check-up. The doctor looked at me and hardly had to touch my belly before he knew. "This baby's breech, we might have a Caesarean delivery here." When I heard that the blood just rushed to my head. I wanted it to be the right way up and come out the right way! The doctor reassured me that a vaginal delivery was still possible and if that was what I wanted, they would do everything they could to ensure a normal delivery. I just went home and cried. When Paul came in I said, "It's upside down the little devil", and he was really upset too. We sat down and looked up Caesarean section in our baby books to get more of an idea – you always skip those pages because you just don't think it's going to happen to you.

It dawned on me suddenly, that if I did have a Caesarean I'd have to have an epidural and the idea of a needle being inserted into my spine terrified me. I wasn't just worried about it, the fear was almost irrational – and yet I didn't want to be put out completely and miss the entire birth. I just kept praying the baby would turn and I spent the entire evening rubbing my belly and whispering, "Come on little one, turn around".

The following day I was making myself a sandwich when I felt this hot trickle in my knickers. I thought, 'Oh God, how disgusting, I've wet myself'. I went to the bathroom and took a look, there was no colour to it, just very hot water. I rang the hospital and told them that I thought my waters were leaking. I was only 36 weeks and they told me to come in straight away. I managed to track down Paul and we made our way there together.

We had to wait ages before we were seen by anyone and I was getting more and more worried. This little baby had been through so much already, I couldn't believe something else could go wrong. Finally, it was confirmed that my membrane had fractured and that meant I was open to infection. Also, if the baby was born now it would be premature and would therefore have to be incubated.

Neither situation was good, but they did consider that if I got through the next 24 hours without going into labour I probably would be okay. I was taken up to the antenatal ward and told to stay in bed. I was very, very frightened. I didn't want the baby to be born if it wasn't ready for it. 'Little one, little one, stay in there, hang on for as long as you can.' I didn't sleep at all that night.

The next morning, three female doctors arrived and said, "Okay, nothing's happened, so we're going to top you up with plenty of fluids and take your temperature three times a day to make sure there's no infection and hopefully that will take you to 37 weeks, when the baby will be older and stronger". Well, I was impressed. I thought, 'Yes, this is good, this is the right thing'.

Everybody was so sweet to me, they gave me a single room so I didn't have to see all the new babies arriving and it gave me a week to prepare myself. I was reading, relaxing and generally having a really good time. The night before I was due to be induced, however, I became really scared. I didn't want to lose my bump, it was quite comfy and I liked talking to it.

The doctor arrived and explained that the following morning they would put some special gel into my vagina and then things would start moving. She did her best to allay my fears but I had quite a lot of trouble getting to sleep. Then at about 1am I woke up with a terrible pain. I knew that feeling. Ten minutes later I got another one, then another at 18 minutes, then another at six minutes. I was in labour! Oh, I was so pleased, my body had done it naturally with no intervention, my baby was ready to be born. The pain was awful, but I didn't care, I felt wonderful and very natural. I called the nurse, who was really pleased too, and she went off to ring Paul. By about 3am the pain was unbelievable. How can you have such a terrible pain and then two seconds later be back to normal?

Paul arrived about 4.15am which helped take my mind off things a bit. As I got a contraction, he would rub my back furiously and it did ease the pain a little. Throughout my pregnancy everyone had said that because I didn't suffer from period pains I would be able to cope much better in labour. Don't you believe it!

At 7am the doctor came to see me. She said there was no need for me to go to the delivery room yet and that I was doing fine. The next few hours were like an eternity; the pain would sweep over me and I would grip Paul for dear life, then it would subside, giving me a few moments to relax and get my breath back. By the time they arrived to take me to the delivery suite at about 12.15pm, I was absolutely gasping for some pain relief.

The suite wasn't what I had expected at all. We'd agreed I should have an epidural in case they needed to do an emergency Caesarean, but unfortunately the lovely birthing rooms which I'd seen on my hospital tour just weren't geared up for it. So I found myself in this horrible room which was all metal and lights and equipment. I got really frightened and tried to hold back the tears but I couldn't.

The midwife was fantastic, she held me in her arms and hugged me and told me over and over again that it would be all right and there was no need to be frightened. I wish I'd been a bit more receptive when the delivery procedures were explained to us at the antenatal classes: you just don't think there'll be any complications when it's your turn. My advice to any expectant mum is to find out about every possible eventuality and then at least you will be more prepared when the time comes.

When they arrived to do the epidural I was petrified. Paul could see how frightened I was and tried to reassure me, but I could see his face as they inserted it and I think he felt it as much as I did. My legs went numb almost immediately and I thought, 'That's it, I'll never walk again'. I knew I was being irrational, but I just couldn't help it. I'd imagined myself walking around, coping with the pain, and of course it was nothing like that. There I was, wired up to a drip and totally confined to the bed; and instead of my body telling me what to do, all these machines had taken over.

After about an hour and a half the epidural began to wear off and I could feel my legs again. I asked them not to top it up too much, I wanted to be able to experience some pain so at least I would feel more in control. A lot of doctors were present because it was breech, but I found them all very caring and supportive. One of the midwives examined me and said, "Oh, that was quick, you're fully dilated". A doctor took over and said, "I can feel what sex it is, do you want to know?" Before I could say no, I had this tremendous urge to push, it really came from deep within my body, "I want to push, I want to push".

The doctor told me to hang on for a second and then said, "I'm sorry, your baby's leg is down by the side of its bottom, we only like to deliver breech babies vaginally when they are in a well-flexed position". My heart sank. "Isn't there anything you can do? They explained that they would try and push the baby's foot up, but if it didn't work they would have to perform a Caesarean. Someone was on my side, because after two or three minutes they managed to do it. I was absolutely delighted and asked if I could start pushing. They said I could once the epidural was topped up.

Suddenly I began to feel really hot and then freezing cold, I could feel myself slipping into unconsciousness. I shouted to them, "Something's wrong, I'm going". They explained that it was my blood pressure dropping and gave me an injection, which brought me back to normality within seconds. Then they said that the baby was in distress and started talking about a Caesarean again. I could feel the baby already halfway down the birth canal and knew that a Caesarean at this stage would be wrong.

They decided to take some blood from its bottom to test whether it was really in distress or not, but they couldn't get enough and it seemed to take forever. I was thinking of every swear word imaginable. Eventually they got enough blood and the results came back that the baby was okay. Then it was action stations. One of the doctors said, "Right, this is it, let's get this baby born".

Suddenly, it was as if I had all the energy in the world. I was so happy and so strong and I thought, 'Yes, this is my baby and I'm going to get it out'. They told me to put my chin down, grab hold of the bars on the bed and go for it. The way I was feeling I could have pushed out a double decker bus because within seconds half my baby was out.

The doctors couldn't believe it. One of them shouted, "*Stop!*... pant, pant... someone take her leg" and then, very quickly, "his leg, its leg". I knew the doctor had let the cat out of the bag, but I just laughed. They cut me so I could deliver her easily and then with two little pushes, she was born. They checked her over very quickly and then put her in my arms. I was just so overwhelmed, tears were pouring down my cheeks – but I was laughing too. I couldn't take my eyes off her, she was so tiny but just so beautiful.

Paul was looking at me and looking at our baby and we couldn't stop laughing, we just couldn't believe it. We'd both been so worried after the miscarriage and when we discovered she was breech and now here she was, healthy and perfect. As I put her to my breast, I closed my eyes and thanked God from the bottom of my heart.

Katie, 33, freelance journalist, and Billy, 42, computer analyst

"Oh, darling, giving birth is just like a bit of backache and constipation"

"There's meconium in the water, the baby's in distress"

"The clock went around and around and around"

I remember going to the loo with the predictor stick, having a pee on it and then, when the line went blue, just screaming, "Aaah!" I was pregnant, wonderful, it was really fantastic.
I felt a bit nauseous at the beginning but was never actually sick. In fact, once, when Billy and I were driving along in the car, I yelled at him, "Stop the car, stop the car, I'm going to be sick", but instead of throwing up I just burst into tears. My emotions were all haywire in those first few months. Also my sense of smell was heightened, I mean I could smell the cat food while I was upstairs, yuk it was horrible, so unless Billy did it, the poor thing never got fed.
I have to admit to being overweight before I got pregnant and so I was really concerned that I would balloon. When I went for my first eight-week check I said to the doctor: "Okay, now I had better go on a diet" only to be quickly told, "Oh no you don't". Well, that was great for me – for the first time in my life I didn't have to worry about being overweight. I was allowed to get bigger without people looking at me and saying, "Tut, tut, she's piling on the pounds".
In fact, I was very careful, and eating really healthy food and keeping active meant that in the end I only put on two stone. I did feel slightly guilty about my smoking, though. I didn't quit altogether, but really managed to cut down. I worked up until 29 weeks and found it virtually impossible not to have the odd cigarette.
I constantly worried about whether my baby would be all right, that was on my mind a lot. One of my assignments during the pregnancy was to cover Fergie visiting a special care baby unit. I remember thinking, 'I can handle this. First of all I'm a journalist and, secondly, I'm a pregnant journalist'… but of course I couldn't. All those tiny

little babies struggling for life, it was so distressing, and made me worry all the more.

However, things went happily on health-wise and I began to think about how I wanted to have the baby. I decided to make it as natural as possible without any pain relief and certainly not an epidural. I had a romantic vision of the pain starting, and of turning to my husband and saying, 'Oh darling, drive me to the hospital, the baby's coming' while he mopped my fevered brow. It took my next-door neighbour, who is a midwife, to bring me gently back down to earth.

Her advice – which I think is the best advice to give any prospective mum – was to keep a completely open mind. Don't think too much beforehand about how you want your labour to be. Too many women are devastated when they plan for a completely natural labour only to find that, for all sorts of reasons, it simply isn't possible. To be honest, it was a relief not to have to work out a detailed birth plan, and I spent the rest of the pregnancy enjoying myself buying all the baby bits and pieces.

I was 40 weeks pregnant when one evening I had an accident in the kitchen. Billy didn't get home from work until ten that night, which meant we were eating later than usual. I was tired and my balance was a bit wonky. I went to the sink to drain a pan of spaghetti and I don't know how it happened, it just seemed to go in slow motion, and the boiling water spilt all over my stomach. I thought, 'Don't panic, don't panic, it can't get to the baby, the baby can't be hurt'. But it was all over me.

I ran into the living room and ripped all my clothes off. Thank God Billy knew what to do. He shoved me back into the kitchen and started throwing loads of cold water over me. The kitchen floor was awash, so I rushed upstairs to the bathroom and held the shower over my stomach, trying not to worry about it, trying to do breathing exercises. Billy dashed off to get the car ready and within minutes we were on our way to casualty.

Thankfully the burn hadn't gone too deep. The hospital staff said it would have been much worse if Billy hadn't had the sense to keep applying cold water. As it was, it was only first degree and of course the baby was fine. The worst part about it was that I had to have the dressing changed every day.

The accident happened on the Friday and the following Wednesday I had an antenatal check. My blood pressure was sky high and the consultant took one look at my stomach and said, "You're being admitted now!" Well, as you can imagine, I was just shaking. "What do you mean, can't I go home at all?" "No." "Well, can I move my car?" "No." Billy wasn't with me and I really began to panic. I tried to find the public phones so that I could ring him and then I couldn't find any change. I was just fumbling around like an idiot, it was awful. Eventually I got hold of Billy, who managed to calm me down, and we organised for him to throw some things into a suitcase for me. Then I had to wait for this rickety little ambulance to take me round to the antenatal ward. They'd rung ahead to let them know I was coming and as I walked in they said, "Ah, the spaghetti lady!"

They were absolutely lovely and showed me to a ward with five other women. Everybody was very friendly and nice, but I found it quite traumatic. From where I was positioned, I could see all these happy mothers being trundled out of the labour rooms with their new babies and after a few days I began to think mine was never going to come. I know it sounds silly, but I started to feel that I was going to be there for the rest of my life.

On the following Monday when still nothing had happened, they decided to induce me. The midwife arrived and pulled the curtains around the bed. I distinctly remember her snapping on these rubber gloves, like some manic surgeon from a horror film. She inserted two pessaries and, oh boy, was it painful. Typically, with the way things were going with me, nothing happened. You see, my baby was determined to be a Leo and we were still in the sign of Cancer! Tuesday came and went and nothing happened. Then, on Wednesday morning at 5 o'clock, hooray! period pains. I went to the loo and saw that I'd had a show and thought, 'Yes, this is it!' I rushed back to the ward as high as a kite and told the midwives what was happening. I was thoroughly disappointed when they said, "No, you're not in labour. A show doesn't mean anything, it could still take days".

For the next three to four hours I coped with the period pains, and then the backache started. At my antenatal classes they suggested that you lean against something and wiggle, which is supposed to relieve the pain. So with each contraction I would start to wiggle, much to the amusement of everybody on the ward. The pain was coming every 15 minutes, but it was bearable and all in my back, nothing in my stomach.

I'd heard about the Tens machine and that you're meant to use it from your first twinge. So, having had one or two twinges by now, I asked the midwife, "Can I have my Tens machine?" She flatly refused, saying, "You're not in labour, just ignore it. If you were at home you'd be doing the housework". Well, it's not easy to ignore it when you're in the middle of an antenatal ward, with pregnant women all around and screams coming from every delivery suite.

I hated being told I wasn't in labour, it got me really angry. I thought, 'Well, if I'm not, then what is this pain and what's happening to me?' Billy arrived, and we started timing the contractions. For a while they would come every five minutes, and then go back to every 10 to 15 minutes. It was getting ridiculous, there was no doubt that something was happening, so Billy and I pinned down a midwife who agreed that she would come and examine me at ten that night.

I went off and had a bath to help me relax. I was coping with the pain but it was beginning to get difficult. My mother had taken five hours to have me and two hours with my brother. My grandmother had twins and she had told me, "Oh darling, giving birth is just like a bit of backache and constipation". So I was under the impression, having spent the last 16 hours in varying degrees of pain, that I didn't have too much further to go.

The midwife arrived on the dot of ten, examined me, and said I was 80 per cent effaced, which meant I hadn't even dilated yet. I can't tell you how I felt, my heart sank. Apparently the cervix has to roll back before it can start dilating and you can be walking around for days like that and not even know. The midwife said, "We'll get you some sleeping pills and you can go to sleep here on the ward and we'll see how you're getting on in the morning".

Well, at that point I just freaked. I burst into floods of tears and by some miracle the labour sister was walking past at that very moment. She marched over, took one look at me and said, "This woman needs to be in the labour room *now!*" *The* relief was immense, at long last I was going into a room of my own; I was going to have some privacy and somebody had finally acknowledged that I was actually in labour. They settled me in and said Billy should go home and they would ring him when it was necessary. Everybody left the room, the lights were turned out and I found myself in pitch darkness.

Thirty seconds later the flood gates opened; my waters had broken. I rang for the nurse in an absolute panic. It was like having your first period; you know one day it's going to happen, but it's a shock when it does. The midwife came running in and quickly sent somebody off to find Billy, who was apparently just walking out of the hospital. As he arrived, I heard the midwife say, "There's meconium in the water, the baby's in distress!" I remember getting hysterical and yelling, "Just cut me open and get my baby out, please make sure my baby's all right!" It was so frightening to hear those words; you don't know enough to understand what's really going on, and I was convinced my baby was in danger.

They calmed me down and gently explained that when I had burst into tears so violently on the antenatal ward, my baby had responded to my distress and also got upset. She assured me that the baby was fine now and not to worry. I pulled myself together and thought, 'Okay, let's get on with this'. I was using the gas and air when the pain got really bad and it seemed to help a lot. It doesn't completely take the pain away but you're so spaced out you couldn't care less anyway. Bugger the bleeding breathing techniques!

By 3am I was only 1cm dilated and realised that I still had a very long way to go. At this rate I knew I wouldn't be able to carry on for much longer and asked for the epidural. Although they hadn't said anything to me about it, they were delighted that I had made that decision because it does help to bring down your blood pressure. Of course what you don't realise is that it takes quite a while to find an anaesthetist.

So for the next hour and half, which was pretty much a blur of contractions, I coped with the pain as best I could. It really felt as though my back was breaking and I remember saying, "I want to die". But I just kept thinking about my baby and somehow you find the strength to keep going.

The anaesthetist finally arrived and I was asked to curl up on the bed – very difficult when you're in so much pain and nine months pregnant. She inserted the epidural and I had the sensation of an icy trickle going into my spine. It seemed to take effect very quickly, but no-one had told me I wouldn't be able to move my legs and that was a very strange feeling.

I remember that at the time I felt very guilty, but now I think that's silly. I feel that the epidural is every woman's right: when you get a headache you take pain relief; when you have an operation you take pain relief; so why should you be made to feel that you're not a proper woman for taking pain relief when you're giving birth?

Because of the burn, they were unable to attach the monitoring machine to me, so the poor midwife spent seven hours, her entire shift, with her hand on my stomach. After the first five hours of having the epidural inserted it began to wear off. I let it go slightly before asking for a top-up because I hated not being able to move my legs and having to be pulled up the bed all the time.

Billy had gone home to try and get some sleep and returned just before daybreak, when I did a very silly thing by letting the epidural go almost completely. As the staff tried to move me on a contraction, I was actually physically sick with the intensity of the pain. I didn't make that same mistake again! One of the sisters applied some acupressure to my wrist to stop the nausea and it really worked.

The hours passed slowly and Billy remembers the clock going around and around and around. I had only dilated by about 1cm, it was all very long and very laborious. The night shift went off and a whole new team arrived, I think I went through about three teams in all. By mid-afternoon the next day I was at last fully dilated.

However, just my luck, the baby was lying back to back, which meant its backbone was on my backbone. They said I couldn't push until the baby had moved down. It was weird because, as the epidural wore off slightly, I could definitely feel its vertebrae against mine.

An hour later, around 4 o'clock, they gave me the go-ahead to start pushing. Billy held my head and on each contraction he would count to ten while I pushed. But he was counting so slowly that I burst out, "Will you bloody hurry up!" So I'm trying to push, push, push and it's so difficult because with the epidural you have very little sensation and can't feel how much work you're doing. They had attached a monitor to the baby's head and Billy said he could see it moving in and out.

I'd been pushing for about an hour when a doctor came in and said, "Look, you've been in labour far too long, I want to help you get this baby out. With your permission I'm going to give you a ventouse extraction". At that moment in time, having gone through so much, I just wanted to make sure my baby was okay and so I agreed immediately.

I was then told that not many people in the hospital had seen this type of delivery and would I mind if a group of students attended the birth. Well, when your fanny's been open to all the world for nearly two days, it seemed like a fairly irrelevant question. I said, "No, go ahead doctor, the more the merrier", and in the end I guess I had more than 20 people standing around me.

I was cut quite heavily, I'll never forget the clunk, clunk of the scissors, but reassuringly there was no pain. The doctor attached the ventouse and while I pushed, she pulled. Suddenly I had this sort of strange slithery feeling and the baby landed on my stomach. I didn't care what sex it was, I just repeated over and over, "Is it all right, is it all right?" They flipped the baby over and said, "It's a girl and, yes, she's fine".

They whisked her off to check that there was no fluid in her lungs. I honestly didn't care that they took her away so quickly, I just wanted them to check everything out. I felt totally overawed and kept thinking, 'It's a baby, I don't believe it'. The way things had been going I wouldn't have been surprised to have had a gorilla or something!

Words really can't describe the emotion you feel at that moment. One minute you have a bump and the next minute a tiny baby, a real live person. They brought her back to me and showed me her little fingers and toes and of course she was perfect – and huge at 9lb 5oz! The smell of her was something else, unlike anything I'd smelled before. It wasn't like perfume, but it was perfume. Although I had just spent 37 hours having her, I looked at Billy and said, "I want five more of these!"

Helen, 32, health visitor and former midwife, and Jarek, 32, computer programmer

"You look at this enormous bump and think about yourself physically and wish there was another route you could take!"

"I remember throwing up in my daughter Kasha's sink, much to her horror"

"I really didn't have a lot of love for the baby inside me"

My first two pregnancies were unplanned and came as a bit of a surprise to Jarek and I, so when we decided to try for a third child I was quite anxious about it. I didn't know how long it would take, but luckily I fell pregnant within two months and we were both absolutely delighted. I was pretty sick for the first three months, which was horrible, I felt really weak and ill. I remember throwing up in my daughter Kasha's sink, much to her horror, and she never lets me forget it.

The sickness lasted for nearly 20 weeks, and it's such a gradual thing when you start feeling better that you're not really aware of it until one day you just realise you haven't been sick for a few days. I continued working until about 28 weeks but I felt awfully tired and had a really rotten back. I kept thinking, 'Oh I must be getting older'. It had been eight years since my first child and five years since the second, so there had been quite big gaps and I realised I'd been a lot younger eight years ago.

I was surprised, because it had been a planned pregnancy, that I didn't feel happier. I didn't feel depressed or anything like that, but it all seemed so much more of an inconvenience. I also felt that I was betraying Kasha by bringing a new baby into our lives. I love Kasha very much and at the time I didn't have a lot of love for the baby inside me.

I wasn't worried about the health of the baby, which is odd because my first child Tomak was born with a brain tumour and died when he was two days old. In some ways I felt I had already been through the worst and if anything was going to go wrong I'd be able to cope with it, no matter what.

I ruminated for a long time over how I wanted the birth to go. I had been a midwife and felt in quite a privileged position having seen so many women give birth. I knew it hurt, and of course I'd already had two children of my own, so I wasn't going to run away from it and I wasn't particularly frightened of it. Mind you, when I got to eight months I panicked a bit; you look at this enormous bump and think about yourself physically and wish there was another route you could take!

As the weeks went by, I thought more and more about having a home birth. My experience with Tomak had obviously been very traumatic and so with Kasha's birth they really wrapped me in cotton wool. Fortunately, she had only taken two and half hours to be born and I assumed that the timing with this baby would be quite similar. I felt that with Kasha I had proved to myself that I could produce a normal healthy baby and deliver it fairly efficiently.

I really didn't want to go into hospital with doctors and midwives I didn't know, and the more I thought about it, the more I decided I wanted to have this baby at home. There wasn't much resistance, except for one doctor who said, "You're not one of those home birth types are you?" I suggested to him that if he had the opportunity to have sex maybe two or three times in his whole life where would he choose to do it, in hospital in full view of everybody or in the privacy of his own home?

And that's how I felt about it. This was very likely to be my last child and I wanted to do it in a situation that I felt was very much under my control. I had a lot of faith in myself and just felt I could do it and it wouldn't be a problem. I was also incredibly fortunate to have a close friend, Joy, who was a community midwife and who was prepared to do the delivery for me. She did most of my antenatal check-ups as well which was really nice because it became a shared thing between us.

Both Tomak and Kasha had been born a week late so when my due date came and went I wasn't in the least bit worried. One evening I was sitting rather uncomfortably with my aching back and when I moved slightly I got this horrible pain. Jarek took absolutely no notice of me, so I dug him in the ribs and said, "You could give me a bit of sympathy when I shout out in pain", but he was far more interested in watching the news. I thought the baby must be lying on a nerve or something so I didn't take much notice of it and went to bed around 11.30.

At 3.15am I woke with a sort of period pain and thought, 'Hmm, this is interesting. I wonder if it will wear off or if it's the beginning of labour'. So I just lay there and half an hour later I got another one, and then another after 20 minutes. They were very spaced out and weren't really painful, I could just feel these really dull, tender aches, like a period pain that you don't moan about but you just think 'ouch'. About 4.20 I felt Jarek stirring beside me and said, "I think we're going to have the baby today". He beamed at me and we both felt a great surge of excitement.

We lay there until about 5 o'clock, and then decided to get up and organise things downstairs in the living room where we had decided to have the baby. The mattress was already in position by the French windows that lead out on to the garden. So we put clean sheets on and brought an armchair down as well. By now my contractions were coming more regularly, about every 15 minutes, and I had to stand and breathe through them. I'd get one very strong one and then two or three very mild ones, so I thought the pain was more in my imagination. It was still quite early, and I didn't want to wake Joy sooner than necessary, so I thought I'd better keep going for as long as I could.

We decided to play scrabble, and I was winning as well, when I got a really strong contraction. I thought, 'Oh sod this, I need someone to rub my back properly' and, since Jarek was fairly useless at that sort of thing, I decided to ring Joy. She had to go to the labour ward first to pick up all the equipment, and arrived at 6.15. Jarek had gone off to the loo and, like most men, always takes a newspaper and is gone for hours, so I went up and let her in. As I opened the door I had to lean against the wall with the pain, so Joy quickly ushered me downstairs and set about massaging my back, which was wonderful.

Jarek went out to the car to bring in all the stuff and I was really amazed because there was so much of it – it practically filled the room. There was a resuscitation unit, oxygen and gas and air cylinders, suction equipment and even an incubator. It took quite a while to unpack and get ready, and every now and then I'd get a fairly heavy contraction, but I just leaned against the wall and breathed fairly strongly through them. It was around 6.50am when Joy said, "I suppose we had better examine you".

It was very amusing, because I could feel her fingers going right down to the back of my vagina. I was thinking, 'Gosh this is really uncomfortable, Joy', so I jokingly said, "Don't you know what you're doing, can't you find my cervix?" and she said, "Of course I know what I'm doing, I've just got very short fingers". I remember thinking, 'Trust me to pick a friend with short bloody fingers to do this delivery'. Eventually she discovered that I was about 8 to 9cms dilated and decided to call the doctor.

The contractions suddenly came on really strongly and I asked for the gas and air. So out came this diddy little cylinder and I thought, 'This is going to be nice'. I took a couple of puffs and got that lovely numbing effect, like you've been knocked in the middle of the head by something quite pleasant. It takes effect after about 30 seconds and you start breathing it in as soon as a contraction begins. I decided that I didn't want to get too dopey so I stopped using it and thought I'd save it until I really needed it.

On the next contraction I went to use it and the bloody thing had stopped working. Joy said, "Don't worry, I've got some more", and ran off to get another cylinder. But the same thing happened again. We went through three and none of them were working. (Later we found out that it had been a fault in the mask and all the cylinders were full.) Joy rang the hospital to have some more cylinders delivered and I thought, 'They won't make it in time, this baby is coming'. I could really feel the head come right down and I was kneeling on the rug when I suddenly thought, 'If my waters go now, it's going to make a real mess'. I asked them to get something and as they placed some plastic sheeting under me my waters just came gushing out.

Joy said I was now fully dilated and that I could push, but somehow I didn't need to, my baby almost came out by itself. I could feel its head and a burning sensation, something I hadn't felt with the other two, and I thought, 'Oh my goodness, I don't want to push this out'. As my contraction went away the head sort of popped back up again and I remember thinking, 'Oh what a nice baby'.

Joy said, "I think just a little push with the next contraction"... but I didn't feel as if I was in control at all. It was as if my body was taking over, and with the next contraction the head was born.

At that moment there was a knock on the door; the doctor had arrived, and there I was, on all fours, with this head between my legs. I asked Jarek to go and let him in but Joy said, "Don't be so silly Helen, if Jarek goes now he'll miss the delivery". So we forgot about the doctor and within seconds Nadia was born.

She was really beautiful, it was so peaceful, and she didn't cry or anything, she went on to the breast instantly; it was wonderful. Joy suddenly remembered the doctor, so Jarek went up to let him in. He wanted to look Nadia over but she was stuck to me like Super Glue and there was no way she was going to let go. He managed to check her over very quickly, and then left. Things were just so peaceful and calm.

Joy, Jarek and I cooed over Nadia, and then we heard Kasha coming down the stairs so Jarek went to meet her and bring her down. It was lovely because she had helped me get the room ready only a few days before and she was still really excited. She came in and said, "I knew it was going to be a girl, oh thank you Mummy, you knew I wanted a little sister". She looked at Nadia and then said, "I do love her but hasn't she got scruffy hair?" Joy and Kasha washed her and Jarek made breakfast for us all. It was a really special time.

I felt so in love with her and all the worries I had during my pregnancy just evaporated. Jarek took Kasha to school and when he got back Joy left. Jarek, Nadia and I climbed into the bed we had made. The sun was shining through the French windows and Jarek and Nadia fell asleep almost straight away. The room was filled with the sound of gentle snoring and I thought, 'The world is a good place to be'.

Lorraine, 36, television producer, and Ron, 37, professional musician

"It was really like two steps forward and three steps back"

"The doctors were literally baying at the door"

"I just wanted my body to tell me what to do"

At the time I was working on a current affairs programme which involved a lot of travelling. I'd been trying to get pregnant for about five months, which isn't very long, but I always seemed to be away at my most fertile time. Ron and I even had a joke about filling up a thermos flask with you-know-what, so I could pack it in my suitcase and whip it out at the appropriate time. You get used to thinking that you can regulate everything, but of course you can't regulate getting pregnant. So when I discovered I was… well, I was absolutely delighted.

I started quite early on being very, very sick. I could be sick everywhere and anywhere, literally. I would be in a shop or a meeting and just have to rush out. In fact, there were only two weeks in the middle of the pregnancy when I wasn't sick. My GP said she had never known anybody like me.

Anyway, one day I was feeling particularly wretched and my Father, who is a strong advocate of yoga, suggested I try it because he believed it would help me. I'd always resisted anything like that: I'm a very fast person and generally do very active things like aerobics or squash to help me wind down. But I was feeling so terrible that day I would have tried anything, so my Father lay me down on the floor and took me through some gentle postures and deep breathing exercises. To my amazement I actually did feel better and from then on I really got hooked. By the end of my pregnancy I was going to three or four classes a week. I found the whole thing totally relaxing and became a much calmer person as a result.

I began reading everything I could about childbirth and was also seriously considering my birth plan. I wanted to do it as naturally as possible, and began practising a yoga squatting position, which tones

75

and strengthens all the right muscles. However, having said this, I still had a very open mind about the whole thing and I certainly didn't rule out the use of pain relief if I needed it at the time. I was very much of the opinion that the pain of labour is a pain that's known to your body. You shouldn't be frightened because you know what's causing it and why you're having it.

Two weeks before my due date, I went along for my normal hospital check-up and I got this bee in my bonnet about wanting to see the consultant. Unless there is a real problem, you don't normally get to see him, but I just felt I had the right to. He was definitely rather impatient with me and obviously thought I was wasting his time. After examining me, he looked up at me over his bifocals and said, "Of course a woman of your size is always going to be a problem. I wouldn't rule out the possibility of a Caesarean". This absolutely floored me. I *am* small, just under 5ft, but nobody had ever mentioned it being a problem before.

I was absolutely furious and felt like I was losing control. I am a professional and used to dealing with people on a professional basis, yet he made me feel very much like 'the little woman'. I came out knowing that I hadn't handled the situation properly, I hadn't asked any questions, hadn't made my feelings clear, I'd just sat there and let this pompous man ride all over me.

I work in a very male-orientated industry and yet, somehow, having this bump in front of me made me lose all sense of who I was. I felt so sure that nature would give me a baby that I could deliver myself. After spending nearly nine months with one idea of how things were going to be, it just seemed so unfair that suddenly I might have to consider looking at it from a different viewpoint. I guess at the end of the day it was the shock of suddenly being told there might be a problem, and I wished the doctor had been a little bit more sympathetic.

That night I was supposed to go to yoga, but I just felt too exhausted and was still upset about what had happened at the hospital. I went to bed and had a good night's sleep, but woke at about 7 o'clock to go to the loo. There was quite a lot of blood around the toilet bowl and, although it didn't frightened me, I thought I'd better ring the hospital anyway. They told me to come in, and when I arrived they weren't sure if it was the show or whether I'd started bleeding, so they kept me in for observation.

That night I was lying in bed tossing and turning and, now this does sound awful, but I just kept thinking I wanted to go for a massive shit! This went on all night and in the morning I told the lady in the bed next to me who said, "Do you think they might be contractions?" This had never actually occurred to me. We decided to time them and discovered they were coming every 15 minutes.

This certainly didn't fit into my plans. I had so much wanted to start my labour at home and stay there for as long as possible. You know, you have all these ideas about going on walks and doing little things around the house to help take your mind off the pain. I kept my fingers crossed that they might let me go home, but it transpired that once you are in hospital for observation they keep you in for 48 hours, so there was no way they were going to let me go.

They moved me to an antenatal ward and by 3pm the contractions were really quite powerful. They monitored me and said I was only in intermittent labour, which is when your contractions stop and then start up again a few hours later, and that this would probably go on for some days. But I had this strange feeling that it probably wouldn't and packed Ron off to get my Evian spray, a bean bag and a homoeopathic tincture called Rescue Remedy, which is very good for shock and stress.

After he had gone, I settled down to listen to some opera on my Walkman. It was *La Boheme* and I had tears of joy running down my face. I felt totally calm and peaceful, I just knew that this was real labour and my baby was going to be born soon. Ron had a gig that night and as the staff insisted that I was still in intermittent labour, it was decided that he could go. But as the afternoon progressed my contractions got stronger and stronger. By 6pm they were so intense I just looked at him and said, "There's no way you're going to do that gig tonight, you're staying here with me because I'm going to give birth".

I put on the Tens machine at this point because I was finding it harder to cope with the pain. I'd been walking around a lot and I really wanted to go for a stroll outside, but the staff refused to let me leave the building. This annoyed me so much that I just sneaked off and got back before they missed me.

I kept trying to squat as I had practised in my pregnancy, but it wasn't easing the pain at all; in fact, it exacerbated the pain in my back. I kept saying to Ron, "I can't work out why it isn't helping... if only my body would tell me what to do".

But I couldn't seem to get that line of communication going. I started to get flustered and went through a few yoga positions until I found that kneeling on all fours and arching my back in a position called 'the cat' eased the pain considerably. From then on I was walking up and down and each time I got a contraction I would drop down on to all fours, which must have been quite a funny sight.

I was coping well at this stage and I found the Tens machine really helped. As the evening wore on, I just went into a complete world of my own. I had no idea what was going on around me, it was like being in a vacuum, just me and the pain. Occasionally, one of the midwives would come and say they would examine me shortly, but for one reason or another they just didn't get around to it.

By 10.30pm I really was in a lot of pain, I hardly seemed to have any time at all between my contractions. Ron was spraying my face with the water and I was sipping the Rescue Remedy, which I found very soothing. Then I started to feel sick and for the first time that night went to lie down on my bed.

There seemed to be no respite from the pain, so Ron and I turned up the Tens machine, but I started to feel the electrical current, which I hadn't been aware of until then. The sensation was really horrible so we turned it down again. I said to Ron, "If I'm only 2cms dilated I'm going to cry because I'm in so much pain". I decided I would definitely have the epidural because there was no way I felt I could cope with it for much longer. For the first time I got really angry and insisted on being examined. The midwife turned up, had a look and said, "My dear, you're 9cms dilated".

Well, that was just fantastic. Ron and I were so pleased, and at that moment my waters broke. I experienced a tremendous relief and this lovely hot liquid flowed down my legs. I was fired with so much energy, I almost ran up to the delivery suite. Once I was settled in I was surprised because I'm normally quite a noisy person but this quiet, very introspective mood came over me.

Ron was wonderful, giving me lots of support without intruding on my concentration. He didn't push himself on me, but just did whatever I wanted, whether it was massaging my back or cooling me down. I don't remember consciously doing anything about the breathing. I think it just happened naturally because I'd practised it so much in yoga. For the next half an hour my contractions subsided and the midwife set about getting ready the things that I had asked for, like a birthing cushion and some gas and air. I could hear other women screaming and shouting, but I didn't feel like that at all, I was actually very calm. I was so thrilled that I had got this far when nobody seemed to think I was even in proper labour and I knew that I only had about an hour to go. Suddenly I got the urge to push and Ron placed the gas and air mask over my face, but it was awful, really claustrophobic, and I flung it away. I seemed to have quite a lot of time between contractions, so after each push I had ten minutes or so to recoup my energy. I already knew that hospital policy was to give you only about an hour of pushing time and when my hour was up I began to get a bit anxious. By 1.30 in the morning the doctors were literally baying at the door ready to give me a forceps delivery, but even though I was tired, I knew I had the strength to go on. I had been sitting mainly in a squatting position on the birthing cushion, but I had a go at standing and doing various other things. I would push, and Ron and the midwife would say they could see the baby's head, but as soon as I stopped it would be sucked right back up. It was really like two steps forward and three steps back.

A doctor poked his head around the door to say, "Look, what shall we do, she's been pushing for long enough". The midwife, who I have to say was absolutely wonderful, just looked at him and said, "This lady is having a baby and she is having her baby in her own good time, so go away". I continued pushing and, although I had decided to tear and not have an episiotomy, I really felt like I was about to burst.

I said to the midwife, "You are going to have to help me". (Ron told me afterwards that she had actually been quietly getting together all the bits and pieces, but she hadn't said anything to me until I'd asked, which again was really good of her.) I don't remember feeling anything at all when she cut me. I gave a few more pushes and suddenly the baby came out. The midwife held up this tiny little thing and said, "Well, what is it then?", which was really lovely because Ron and I had so wanted to discover the sex of the baby for ourselves. I remember him saying, "Oh, it's a girl". He was ecstatic and burst into tears.

79

I know this sounds a bit odd, but I wasn't that interested in her; she was crying, and Ron took her. It was weird, I was like a detached observer and he just looked at her with so much love and she looked at him and I realised this was the beginning of a love affair.

I wasn't really aware of anything except this great sense of relief; my baby was here and she was okay. They moved me to my room and that night I put her in the nursery because I felt I needed some time on my own.

The following morning I awoke with a start and felt this terrible gap, 'Where was my baby!' The urgency to get her was all-consuming; only a few hours earlier I hadn't been that bothered, but now I desperately wanted her. I rushed to the nursery and brought her back to bed with me. I was hugging her when Ron walked into the room and said, "Roses for my two girls". There he was, with two enormous bouquets, one for me and one for our little daughter Lenneke.

Janine, 24, ceramic artist, and Dan, 27, mature student

"I bet you'll be one of those people who has a water birth"

"It was like a knife going into my vagina and being twisted around"

"Nobody tells you how beautiful the smell of a newborn baby is"

Well, I wasn't married and at first I was frightened. I told my boyfriend, Dan, and he just said, "Great, that's no problem, we'll get married". That made me feel really positive and I suddenly realised, yes, it is great, I'm going to have a baby. Up until then, although I was 21, I think I was still trapped in a 16-year-old frame of mind. But I suddenly realised I quite old enough to handle it and it didn't seem such a big deal. It was the 1990s after all and, together, Dan and I would cope with the situation. From then on, we were both really excited.

I started to feel special, something wonderful was happening to me. I hadn't really thought about how I wanted to have the baby but friends started saying, "Oh, I bet you'll be one of those people who has a water birth". The idea really appealed to me, because I adore the water, but I thought it would be far too expensive, and put the idea out of my mind.

Soon after this we moved to Newport and I registered at the local hospital. I was herded in and out with all the other pregnant women and suddenly this feeling of being so special began to evaporate and I felt like I was on a conveyer belt. I remember that night I was almost in tears when Dan got home. I explained what had happened, how unimportant I felt and Dan, in his normal brilliant way, said, "Okay, if you don't want to go back to the hospital you don't have to, we'll organise for the midwife to come and see you".

It was at this point that we heard about an organisation called Birthworks who are based in Plymouth. They specialise in natural childbirth and, after chatting to them, we discovered that a water birth was actually not that expensive and Birthworks could arrange everything for us. Dan and I were absolutely over the moon because, for us, this seemed the perfect solution.

The pregnancy was progressing normally, but because we were in a new house I didn't know anybody in the area, and I found it increasingly difficult to fill the day until Dan got back from college. I just used to lie down on the sofa eating and I put on around four stone! I was so lethargic and couldn't coax myself into doing anything. Finally I phoned Birthworks and they were really helpful and positive. The woman I spoke to suggested taking up swimming and this just seemed so logical. I was going to have a water birth, so what better way to help myself and my baby to prepare for the big day.

I went off to Mothercare, bought myself a swimsuit, got out my bike and, from then on right up until the birth, I swam at least three times a week. I began to feel really fit and healthy. It just completely changed my life and every time I went I imagined what it would be like to give birth in the water. As the weeks went by I became more and more excited.

My due date eventually came and went. I was ten days late when the midwife said, "You're going to have to be induced if the baby doesn't come within the next few days". The prospect of this was awful. The tank had arrived and was sitting in our kitchen ready and waiting. Suddenly we were faced with the possibility of having to go into hospital and our carefully laid plans would all go out the window.

I was really annoyed because I'd tried everything: eating rhubarb and plates of curry; seven-mile bike rides; and swimming more frantically than ever. With some desperation I asked the midwife if there was anything else I could do. It was very funny, because she was quite prim and proper, and she lent over and whispered in my ear, "Well dear, you know sex can work wonders".

We'd been having sex right the way through, but she explained that it wasn't the physical act, but actual chemicals in the semen that can help bring on contractions. So that night we went to bed and said, "Let's try for a baby!" I must say it was very mechanical, but amazingly I started to have contractions.

I didn't tell Dan at first because I thought by saying it, it wouldn't be true. The pain was very mild, almost undetectable, but coming regularly every five to six minutes. Eventually I told Dan, and we went downstairs.

It was like a party, we were giggling, messing around and just so excited. Dan started to fill the tank because it takes about two to three hours and I was sitting sewing, trying to take my mind off it, when the midwife arrived. Between contractions we were taking photographs, juggling and playing games. I don't think she quite knew how to take it.

Things began to get more serious after a while. The contractions were suddenly getting very strong and I can't tell you how great it was to have Dan there. He was my point of focus, because you need something to concentrate on through the pain. If he wasn't looking straight at me and breathing with me, because he was saying something to the midwife, I'd grab his head and turn it towards me so that I could look into his eyes again. It was weird, because the pain would intensify even if he looked away for just a second, which I was really suprised at.

Dan rubbed my back and I leant on him for support. The midwife examined me and estimated that I'd probably be about another hour, and it was at that time that I felt I wanted to be in the water. I remember having this sudden flash image of me standing on the kitchen sideboard and diving in, and I couldn't stop laughing. I went into hysterics and Dan and the midwife were wondering what I was laughing about.

I found sitting in the tank really comfortable because the pressure on my abdomen was lifted instantly and I think the baby recognised the feeling of being in the water because I'd swam so much throughout my pregnancy. Dan had to kneel behind me and hold me up, otherwise I found it difficult to remain still. The tanks are actually quite big and you find yourself floating around if you're not careful.

At first everything seemed to be going quite smoothly. The second midwife had arrived, because you have to have two present for the birth, and we were all expecting the baby to come fairly soon.

However, it just seemed to go on and on, the pain was intensifying, and I remember thinking, 'This is getting really serious'. I began to see in black and white literally and was actually going under the water from time to time. I got to the classic stage of wanting to give up, all I wanted to do was sleep. I was so tired by then and had just about had enough.

The midwife got quite stern and shouted at me, "Come on now, wake up, let's get this baby delivered". She wanted to give me an internal examination and also to break my waters because the labour had been going on for too long. I sensed a real urgency about it and, although I didn't want anyone to touch me, I let her carry on. It was incredibily painful but once she had done it the relief was immense and I could actually feel the baby begin to move down. It was such a weird sensation, like having a big poo, the biggest in your life, and nowhere in any of the books does it say anything like that.

My eyes were closed and I felt like I was just a head, a stomach, and a leg on each corner, with this massive thing coming down straight from my heart. I could feel the baby's head moving down inch by inch and I instinctively knew it was time to push. Then this amazing thing happened: as I pushed, an even bigger push seemed to come from inside me, it was as if I was getting outside help. I felt as if my body was doing all the work for me. I had this terrible stretching feeling, God it was awful, but after 17 hours at long last I knew that something very positive and exciting was about to happen and that helped to override the pain.

As my baby's head came through I experienced the most dreadful pain of all. It was like a knife going straight into my vagina and being twisted around. I screamed and the screams came through me from nowhere. The midwife told me to calm down; I did feel at this point that I was losing control and it was only her authoritarian manner that brought me back together again. When the baby's head came out the cord was twisted around its neck, but the midwife was so professional that I didn't panic – she just dealt with it very quickly. I gave a final push and Lucien was brought up to the surface.

From then on it was complete ecstasy. Dan and I were both crying and I remember saying, "Dan talk to him, he knows your voice". He was all wrinkly and purple, just so soft, I couldn't get over how soft he was. Nobody tells you how beautiful the smell of a newborn baby is. The smell is so sweet and, considering this baby had just come from my insides, it amazed me that he smelt so good – and for days afterwards too.

His eyes were so bright and so shiny and from the moment he was born he just looked around, totally alert. I had this tremendous feeling of unity, we were a family now. He didn't cry once and from that moment on I didn't let him go.

Jane, 35, freelance art director, and David, 35, classical violinist

"I had my second scan and I clearly saw this little thing wipe its nose"

"I was sitting on the toilet at 7.05pm when my waters broke"

"I was having contraction on contraction"

It was Christmas-time when I met David. He only lived two doors away and we fell instantly in love. It was a typical whirlwind romance and in the April he asked me to marry him. We discussed having children from the onset really – I was 34 and knew time was ticking away. So, thinking it would take us at least two years to get pregnant, we didn't bother to use any contraception.

David had to go away on business and I can remember feeling totally irrational about it. My period was late and I put it down to pre-menstrual tension and the fact that I was missing him so much. I was redecorating the bathroom and I ended up sobbing on the floor, just sobbing my heart out, I found I couldn't cope with anything.

I began to wonder if I could possibly be pregnant and when David came back we did a test. Not surprisingly, it was positive, and we were both absolutely elated. Because of David's business commitments we couldn't arrange to get married until August, by which time I was 17 weeks pregnant. I was already beginning to show and at each fitting the wedding dress would have to be let out!

Before I got pregnant I was never really the maternal type. I loved my sister's kids, although they were probably the first kids I'd ever loved. But I had never been interested in babies and I became terribly worried that I wouldn't love my own. I'd recently been made redundant and had set up my own business working from home. I was suddenly terrified that it would all be too much for me. I'm a terribly disorganised person and I wasn't sure that I'd be able to cope. Physically I was very fit, but I did get terrible problems with constipation and even the obsessive craving I developed for platefuls of curly kale didn't help to get things moving! On the whole, though, I had a great pregnancy. I couldn't have got depressed if I'd tried. I was just so happy with David, I'd been on a high since the day I met him and life was fantastic.

I booked in with my local hospital and then got in a total panic because all the antenatal classes were full and I had visions of going through the entire pregnancy totally unprepared for the big event. After an awful lot of juggling they were finally able to accommodate me, but from then on I found their approach to my pregnancy quite disappointing.

I thought they'd take more care of you, give you more tests and things. It seemed to me that nobody really gave a stuff. With so many people having babies, mine wasn't important to anybody – except me – and I did resent that. In retrospect, I now realise that it was because I had such a bog-standard pregnancy; whereas a friend of mine who had a lot of problems was monitored constantly.

At 23 weeks I had my second scan, which was terribly exciting. I clearly saw this little thing wipe its nose, and knew instantly that she was a girl – although of course I didn't know for sure. I felt very much that I wanted to have a natural birth. I don't take drugs of any kind, not even aspirin, and I was determined not to take any during my labour. I believe that your body is designed for giving birth and that, unless something goes wrong, you are unlikely to produce a child that's too big to come out on its own. I also feel that modern practices probably prevent you from having a natural childbirth easily.

In the last few weeks of my pregnancy the pressure on my bladder was just awful. I'd end up going to the loo at least four or five times a night. One day I had been energetically wallpapering the hall and fell into bed that night absolutely exhausted. Then at 4.30 in the morning I woke up for one of my frequent trips to the toilet and was terrified to see a mass of bright red blood.

My first thought was that I must be losing the baby. David rang the hospital immediately and was told that there was nothing to worry about, it was just a 'show'. I calmed down and went back to bed, although I was still worried because I'd always been led to believe that a 'show' was just a plug of mucusy stuff, and the sight of all that bright red blood had really petrified me.

David went off to work that morning as usual and my sister came over to help me tidy up the flat, which was in chaos. I knew that things could happen any time now but, apart from the odd twinge, I didn't have any contractions; yet I felt excited the entire day. I was sitting on the toilet at 7.05pm when my waters broke. I knew the time exactly because *The Archers* was on the radio and I missed it.

I rang David and asked him to come home and five minutes later the contractions started. I was pouring water everywhere and had wedged this enormous bath towel between my legs to try and stop the flow. My neighbour was there and my sister, and between us we were having quite a good laugh.

The contractions were coming every five minutes so they were fast right from the beginning; the pain wasn't bad, just a sort of cramping sensation. We'd hired a Tens machine, so we read the instructions and strapped it on. I was in a really good mood, full of fun, and got on the phone to tell all my friends that I'd be giving birth soon.

I didn't want to phone the hospital too early because I had this great fear of being stuck in a room with six other women, lying there for hours and hours, which filled me with absolute horror. By the time we did go in, the contractions were really fast and I went straight to the delivery room. I still had the Tens machine on, which I found brilliant. I kept pressing the button at the wrong moment because I was so overwhelmed by the contractions, so David took over. I'd say, "They're coming, they're coming", and he'd press the button, so that worked quite well.

To my surprise a very nice, rather handsome young man turned up and said, "Hello, my name's Steve, I'm your midwife and how would you like to give birth?" I was a bit taken aback but told him, "I want a completely natural birth and I'd also like to kneel". He said, "That's fine with me, I'd love to do a natural childbirth", which threw me as I was expecting him to say something like, 'Well, we'll do what we can for you dear, but we'll have to see how we get on'.

He examined me and said he thought I was about 3cms dilated but he wasn't sure because I was having quite a strong contraction at the time. A few minutes after this my Mum and sister turned up, which was great because we were all chatting away and it helped to take my mind off the pain.

It was all suddenly spoilt by the arrival of the senior midwife who took one look around the room and said, "What's this then, an appreciation society". I thought it was such a negative thing to say because the pain was really appalling and I needed all the help I could get. Anyway, they were ushered out of the room and she gave me another internal examination.

I was mortified when she told me that I hadn't even begun to dilate and I wouldn't be giving birth for ages. The pain was beginning to overwhelm me; I was trying desperately to breathe through the contractions and to stay calm, but all this did was to send me into a complete panic, thinking, 'How am I going to cope?' The senior midwife wanted me to go back to the labour ward, but it was full so we ended up in a little private room of our own. I found out later that Steve the midwife had told my Mum that he didn't think it would take too long at all, but since he was a junior there was nothing he could do.

By now it was the middle of the night and we decided to put some music on. David is a violinist and had recorded a piece called *Lark Ascending* where the music rises and falls rhythmically. The violin seemed to accompany my contractions and it was just so interesting and calming to lisen to. We stayed there, just David and me, and by this time I was really in a lot of pain. Now I was finding it really horrible and the whole novelty thing was definitely wearing thin. The contractions were constant, no sooner had one finished than another one started, and I thought, 'I can't stand this for much longer'. I was beginning to think I'd need an epidural… nobody came to see us, we were totally alone, and I decided to have a bath in the hope that it would ease the pain.

I'd been standing for most of the time and now lying back in the bath seemed to make things worse. Something was obviously happening because I was suddenly bleeding quite heavily. It was absolute agony, such appalling pain I just wanted to die. A number of times I completely lost control and my breathing went to pieces. I think breathing is the secret of childbirth because as soon as you lose that concentration, the pain intensifies even more. You just start wriggling and complete panic takes over.

After five minutes of being in the bath I had a really strong desire to push. I thought, 'This is ridiculous, I've got to have some help'. I was screaming at David, "I want to *push*, I want to *push*, but I knew that you mustn't if you're not ready and I didn't know if I was ready or not. I could feel my body starting to go involuntarily, I couldn't bear it any longer and told David to push the panic button.

When the nurse eventually arrived I told her how strongly I wanted to push and she explained that I wasn't due to have an examination until 4.30am. It was only 2.30 and I knew I couldn't cope with another two hours. She offered to get me some Pethidine and David butted in with, "No, she doesn't want any drugs". I literally screamed, "F... you David, get me some pain relief". If I'd been in the delivery room I would definitely have used the gas and air. This was just too much for me to bear, I couldn't stand it any longer and asked for a mild epidural.

We gathered up our things and made our way to the delivery suite on the next floor. I was having contraction on contraction. I must have woken up a lot of people in the wards because I couldn't stop myself crying out with the pain. As we got out of the lift I had such a massive desire to push that I couldn't walk at all. I was trying so hard not to, but it was impossible.

Somehow I managed to get into the room and Steve, who fortunately hadn't gone off duty, helped me up on to the bed. I was soaking wet and doubling up with the contractions.

Steve managed to feel inside me and said, "You're fully dilated, you can push". I was so stunned by the fact that I was ready and what I had been feeling inside was right. I got into a kneeling position and held on to David.

Steve said he would deliver me from behind and that the baby would fall on to the bed so that I could pick it up straight away. I found the pushing bit horrible, I hated it. It was like having food poisoning, diarrhoea and sickness all at once, a complete involuntary evacuation of the body.

On each contraction you're supposed to push three times, but I found it so unbelievably awful that on the third push I couldn't do it. It's a completely different sort of pain, like a burning sensation at the end of your cervix. I didn't want to push because I couldn't bear the feeling of this thing inside me coming out.

Steve told me he could feel the head, I was nearly there. I was screaming, "I can't bear it", but I gave one almighty push and the baby's head came out. I couldn't believe I wasn't completely torn to pieces, there was this horrendous burning sensation tingling all over my vagina, and then, on my next contraction, out she plopped.

I picked her up and held her in my arms for what seemed like ages before Steve weighed her or anything. David cut the cord and I thought it was the most disgustingly scrunchy noise in the whole world.

It was an amazing sensation seeing her for the first time. She was tiny, only 6lbs, her skin was almost purple and she had such a funny little screwed-up face. I was fascinated by her, and David and I fell instantly in love with her. It was the most painful experience of my life, but it hasn't put me off. Next time round I think I'd like to have a home birth.

Nicola, 25, sales assistant, and Mark, 29, fireman

"I could feel my body just pushing this baby out"

"Basically you're so unconfident that if they told you to hang from the chandelier you'd do it"

"She came at me with this long needle type thing"

Getting pregnant was a complete accident. I was a couple of days late and there wasn't any real reason for it that I could see. The only possibility was that one night the condom had come off inside me, but I really didn't think there was anything to worry about. After a while I found I needed to get up in the middle of the night to use the loo and it was at that time, in the back of my mind, I began to think, 'Oh dear'. My period still hadn't come, so eventually I decided to do a pregnancy test.

It was one of those double ones and the first test went bright pink. I was convinced it was wrong; surely I couldn't be pregnant? I'd done the test in the evening so I thought, 'Well I've done it wrong anyway, as the instructions said first thing in the morning'. When it went pink again, I still didn't believe it and ended up doing about four more. I spent a fortune on the damn things.

In the end I went to my doctor, still convinced that there had to be another reason why my period was late. I told her about the tests and that each one was positive, but that I wanted her confirmation. She said that over-the-counter kits were just as effective as anything she could do, and promptly set about organising my first hospital visit. It really wasn't until the bumf from the hospital arrived that I finally started to believe it.

Then I panicked. I wasn't married at the time and although my relationship with Mark was very good, we'd only known each other for a year or so. I felt like a rat in a cage, as though someone had nailed my tail to the floor. At the time I didn't know if Mark was the man for me and the last thing I wanted was a baby.

91

This may sound a bit weird, but during all this chaos my sister was seeing one of these psychic kind of people, the ones who can tell you what's wrong with your body. I had a thyroid problem, and although I didn't want the baby, I certainly didn't want there to be anything wrong with it. So I gave this woman a call and she basically told me that I would lose the baby. Well, that was it, my whole attitude turned round and suddenly I desperately wanted to have it.

When Mark found out, he was absolutely thrilled, really excited. He had wanted to marry me anyway, so in that respect I was very lucky as he could have packed his bags and disappeared over the horizon. I worried the whole time about what the psychic had said and was convinced that I would miscarry. As the months went by it actually got worse, because if I did lose it, it would be a proper baby and not just an early pregnancy. So I always tried to stay one step back from it; if it was going to happen there was nothing I could do about it.

I don't know how Mark put up with me in those first few months. I was very difficult to live with, really aggressive and unloving, because my hormones were playing havoc. Fortunately this only lasted for the first four months and after that I just got happier and happier. Physically I was absolutely fine, except for mid-term, when I contracted a stomach bug. It frightened the life out of me because it made me so violently sick, but otherwise I was very healthy. I did put on a lot of weight, but as my stomach had been a bit on the big side beforehand, I hadn't seen my thighs for some months anyway, so I didn't worry too much about it.

The irritating thing about being pregnant was that everyone I came into contact with kept touching my bump. I found it very intrusive and remember one occasion when, at a party, an old friend of mine came charging towards me and literally clamped his hands on to my stomach. He at least had the decency to say, "You don't mind, do you?" to which I replied, "Not if you don't"… and promptly grabbed his balls.

I was terrified about how much the labour was going to hurt and wanted it to be as pain-free as possible. The idea of forceps and the inevitable stitches 'down there' was too awful to contemplate. I talked to a lot of people but nobody really wants to tell you the truth to your face. I'd always get, 'Oh, it wasn't too bad', but all I believed was that it did hurt and that it was going to no matter what I did.

I remember watching all the other women in the antenatal classes practising squatting because rumour had it that it was a good way to avoid having stitches. I gave it a go, but found it really tiring, and in the end decided to wait and see what happened on the day.

The baby was due on the 8th February and all day nothing happened. I began to think, 'Well that's it, it's going to be weeks now' and got very bad tempered and fed up. To top it all I was terribly constipated, so that night I took about three laxatives. At one in the morning I woke up with a terrible pain in my stomach, went to the toilet and it seemed like the whole world fell out of my bottom. I had terrible cramp and thought, 'Oh well, I've obviously upset my stomach with the laxatives'.

Fifteen minutes later I was on the loo again. I felt sick and the cramping was pushing down into my stomach but I didn't for one minute associate it with labour. This went on until about three in the morning when I suddenly realised that the pains had a regular pattern to them. They were coming every 15 minutes. Mark got really excited and said, "Maybe you're in labour", but I said, "Don't be silly, I've just got an upset stomach". But by 4am they were coming every seven minutes and by 6am every three minutes. I put on the Tens machine and I don't know if it helped ease the pain, but it did help to distract me. The pain wasn't unbearable, just very uncomfortable, like a sharp cramp.

I wanted to put off calling the hospital because I didn't want to make a fuss but Mark convinced me, and they told us to come in straight away. By the time we arrived, at around 7.15am, the contractions were coming thick and fast. The actual duration of the pain wasn't that long but they were quick, so I wasn't getting much respite. I went straight to a delivery suite and I remember thinking how horrid it was. It seemed so cold and unfriendly and I had to wait there for ages before they finally examined me. When they told me I was only a thumb's nail dilated, I was absolutely gobsmacked.

This was terrible news, I couldn't believe it. They had strapped me up to a monitor when I arrived and the midwife could see that the contractions were quite hard. She was fairly certain that the baby would be born by noon, so that gave me something to focus on and I felt I could deal with another five hours.

The lady in the next room was wailing and screaming. It really shook me up and I burst into tears. The midwife said it would probably be better if I did something to take my mind off it and suggested I go and have a bath.

That was a good idea because it really helped, the pain seemed to be a lot easier, although the contractions were still coming every three minutes. I really thought I was making progress, but when they examined me again at 11am, I still wasn't moving dilation-wise and it was then I realised that the baby wasn't going to arrive by mid-day. For some reason my contractions slowed right down and began to come every six to seven minutes, so I was sent to one of the labour wards. This really depressed me and I felt like a complete failure. I lay on my bed for the next couple of hours, trying to cope with the pain, while Mark read a newspaper.

Suddenly a massive contraction hit me at around 1.30pm and then everything speeded up again. They went back to every three minutes again and the pain was so awful it was like having gastroenteritis. I couldn't lay still and had to get up and walk around. I tried to do my breathing, which was a distraction, something to concentrate on. I was quite upset by now and finding it difficult to cope. Then at 3pm they came to examine me: I was about 4cms dilated and they decided it was best if we went back to the delivery suite.

By now I was actually getting quite tired and beginning to lose heart. I wondered how long it was going to go on. For a while it was just Mark and I alone in the room together. He was really wonderful, helping me with my breathing, but by now the pain was really getting too much for me. I was semi-delirious and relied on Mark an awful lot to be my voice and say what I wanted. Basically you're so unconfident that if they told you to hang from the chandelier you'd do it. Thankfully, Mark asked if there was something they could do to help with the pain and I was given a shot of Pethidine. It made me very sleepy, quite drugged and almost slightly drunk. So in a way I did relax a bit, but it certainly didn't help with the pain and from that point of view I didn't think it was very good.

At 5pm I was still only at 5cms so the midwife said she was going to break my waters to help speed things up. She came at me with this great long needle type thing and I thought, 'Oh my God'. I was having this almighty contraction and begged her to wait until it had passed. I don't know whether it was total fear or not but suddenly my waters broke of their own accord. I just remember feeling this incredible release of warm water, and then things really began to hot up.

The women in our family have a history of taking ages to get to 5cms and then it just goes and we can do the rest in about half an hour. I kept saying this to the midwife but she didn't really take me seriously. I remember yelling at her, "Look, it happened with both my sisters and my Mum and she's had nine kids".

I was squeezing Mark's hand to death and really becoming hysterical. The contractions were just coming too fast for me to cope with, and all of a sudden I got this incredible urge to push. I could actually feel the baby coming down.

I was terribly frightened of the fact that I mustn't push if things weren't ready. The fear was almost more than the pain. The sensation didn't go away. I was screaming, "I can't stop myself, I'm pushing, I'm pushing. Please, please check me now, I know I'm ready". The midwife said, very calmly, "It's all right, just breathe, try not to push. The last time we checked you, you were only 5cms, you can't possibly have dilated so quickly".

The urge got stronger and stronger until it completely overwhelmed me. I could feel my body just pushing this baby out. I was totally out of control, and none of the midwives were helping me, it was terrible. But I just kept going on and on at her to check me and in the end she agreed.

She put her hand inside me right in the middle of a contraction and the pain was like nothing on earth. I let out an almighty scream, it was blood-curdling. I'd never heard myself scream like that. The midwife looked really surprised and said, "Yes, you are ready to go. Push, push". I can't describe how relieved I was to hear those words. I felt like saying, 'Why didn't you listen to me. It's my body, not yours and I know what it wants me to do'.

They turned me on to my side; by now all thoughts of squatting had gone completely out the window. The midwife held on to my legs and it was great because although it was painful, I was going with the pain and not fighting against it. You are taught in class to give three pushes on each contraction. I always thought that sounded ridiculous but it's true. You get a contraction, push, hold it, push, hold it and then push again. I was pushing madly through my bottom, which I'm sure is wrong, but it just seemed the natural thing to do. Mark started shouting that he could see the head, he was getting over-excited but I was like a robot, totally absorbed in what I was doing.

I was pushing as hard as I could but I just couldn't get the head out, so the midwife said she would have to do an episiotomy. It didn't hurt at all and then I remember her getting terribly sort of serious. She said, "Right, now on the next push you're going to get the head out and you must hold it while we check everything". I thought, 'Gosh this is serious', so I did the push and the head came out, which burnt like hell. Then there was a terrible panic because it had the cord around its neck. The midwife was saying, "Stop, stop for God's sake, don't push".

Within seconds they'd untied the cord, clamped it, and suddenly the baby was out. Mark's eyes filled up instantly and I can remember him saying, "Oh my God this is so wonderful". They put the baby straight on to my chest and covered it with a blanket. We took a peek and discovered that we'd got a little baby girl. I didn't feel much emotion myself, I suppose because I was just so exhausted. The whole experience had been so mind blowing, I felt numb.

It wasn't until the following morning that I was able to take it all in, and then I just got so happy, so exhilarated. All the blood vessels on my face had burst, which gives you some indication of the pushing power, and I looked as though I had smallpox. Also, I was doing rather a good impression of John Wayne each time I went to the loo! But none of it mattered, that day I was Mother of the Year.

Barbara, 33, sculptress, and Phillip, 40, freelance film cameraman

"At 33 I just desperately needed to become a mother"

"The creation of a child within my body was a phenomenal feeling"

"These can't be contractions, I would know if these were contractions"

We had been thinking for quite some time about having children, but for me far more than Phillip. I seemed to have a very strong physiological need, a yearning within my body to have a baby. Although I didn't think about it constantly, it was a very big factor in my life at the time. My work was going fine, but at 33 I just desperately needed to become a mother. When I look back now, I can't believe that those emotions were so strong.

Phillip had just gone freelance in the film business and would have preferred to establish himself a bit more before starting a family. We had endless discussions about it before finally deciding to go ahead. Then it all happened very quickly – I was pregnant within a month. From the moment I did the test and found it was positive I felt completely different. Although I couldn't see it or feel it yet, I knew something had happened within my body.

At about eight weeks, the physical changes started, and I got the usual early morning sickness. I was working as a film camera assistant at the time and I remember arriving in the mornings while everyone was tucking into their bacon butties, and doing a quick U-turn because the smell revolted me. I didn't tell anyone at work that I was pregnant apart from the cameraman I worked under. He was really sweet about it, and wouldn't let me carry any of the heavy gear.

Along with working, I carried on riding my horse until around seven months, when I suppose I literally couldn't get on or off it. I discussed it with my doctor from the safety point of view, and he assured me that the actual physical act of riding couldn't do any harm and that only a very serious fall could be dangerous to the baby. As I had been riding all my life I felt the risk was very small indeed.

The one thing that annoyed me about being pregnant was how rapidly my mental capacity diminished. I'd walk into a room and wonder why I'd gone in there; I was forever retracing my steps. It was so frustrating! And, as I got bigger, people began to treat me differently. I was no longer an individual person who had been capable of carving out a career for herself; in their eyes I had metamorphosed into a 'mother' whose only role in life was to look after her baby. It made me feel like a second-rate citizen, and I still fight against that sort of thing now.

I religiously read all the pregnancy books – which I found incredibly exciting – to understand at each stage the changes that were taking place. The creation of a child within my body was a phenomenal feeling. Having said that, I didn't particularly enjoy my body getting bigger, and towards the end I became so huge I was quite sure that my bellybutton, which seemed to be the most vulnerable part of me, would rupture at any minute.

I wanted to have the baby as naturally as possible, and by that I meant I didn't want any severe medical intervention unless it was absolutely necessary. It was very important to me to be totally conscious so I could be part of the whole process.

The first inkling I had that I was going into labour was waking at 2am with slight stomach cramps. They were very slight and in no specific area. I remember thinking, 'These can't be contractions, I would know if these were contractions'. I lay in bed for a while and gradually I realised there was a sequence and it was not random indigestion or stomach rumblings.

I woke up Phil saying, "Look, I think I might be going into labour, but I'm not sure because I don't know what it's meant to feel like!" So we measured the intervals between the cramps and it was like a minute or something. They weren't at all painful, just like little waves rippling through my body. It was very gentle actually, quite pleasant even – and I remember thinking that contractions were supposed to hurt!

We got up and, because you are not allowed to eat anything once you get to the hospital, Phil made me an enormous plate of scrambled eggs. I spent the rest of the morning wandering around the house trying to remember everything I'd been taught.

We suddenly realised that we didn't have a single photograph of me pregnant so we took the opportunity to take some. There was me, proudly posing with my bump, and every now and then we'd stop as I felt another wave come over me. We stuck some music on and I kept thinking, 'I must keep mobile so that I dilate evenly', and all the rest of the things we had been taught in class.

By 5pm the contractions were starting to get a little sharper. They still weren't painful, but they were enough to stop me physically doing anything other than concentrating on this feeling in my body. Because they were stronger, I suggested to Phil that we should go to the hospital.

I went straight to the delivery suite and, after my blood pressure was taken, I was introduced to the team of midwives who had been allocated to me. I had an internal and was amazed to find I was already 7cms dilated. I thought, 'Wow! This is easy'.

After a while, I began to feel very self-conscious just sitting on the end of the bed with Phil and two midwives staring at me, waiting for me to do something. I hated it, it was like being centre stage. For the next hour we chatted idly on every inane subject under the sun. Very stupidly, I didn't follow my instincts to be more mobile. I just assumed the midwives knew more than I did so I stayed on the bed. When they examined me again I hadn't dilated any further, so they suggested breaking my waters. I wasn't sure, but they said it would probably speed things along a little bit. In retrospect, I think this was my biggest mistake.

The baby was quite high up in my womb and with the release of the waters it was suddenly forced down on to my cervix. Its heartbeat started speeding up considerably and they called in the chief midwife. They all huddled together in the corner, which was awful because I didn't know what they were talking about, and then the chief midwife explained they were going to attach a foetal monitor to the baby's head.

I hated the thought of my baby having a clip put on to its skull, but equally if my baby was at risk I knew it had to be done. Although there was only a tiny wire coming out of me, in my mind it felt like a rope was strapping me down to the bed, and I felt if I moved I would damage the baby. It was like being straight-jacketed.

The contractions began to get faster and more severe so I started using gas and air. I don't really remember pain, just overwhelming emotion and my body doing something involuntarily. I remember being very polite to everybody. Apparently, if you are the type to swear and make a fuss in everyday life you become quite reticent and quiet in labour, while women who are normally quiet swear like troopers. Well, as a camera assistant working mainly with men, I did swear a lot, so it seemed the old saying was true.

I kept on thinking this must be awful for Phil, watching me making the most horrible facial contortions with the pain and not being able to help. When they next examined me I hadn't dilated evenly, and I felt this was because I hadn't kept mobile. I began to have an overwhelming desire to push but they told me I couldn't because I would tear. I thought, 'Oh God! Tearing's even worse than not being able to push', and I clenched my fists to stop myself with every contraction. I thought, 'If we are meant to have babies why is it so bloody difficult?'

More people were whizzed in and suddenly it seemed like Clapham Junction. I just wanted it to be nice and quiet but then they said, "Okay, we can try pushing and see how we go". It was the most wonderful relief in the world; I started putting all the energy I had been storing up into pushing. Suddenly there were shouts of, "Stop, stop, stop". The baby's heart rate had dropped and was dropping rapidly. All hell broke loose and it was Emergency Ward Ten.

I knew something was seriously wrong, I wanted them to get the baby out. I didn't care how, they could have cut me open there and then as long as the baby would be okay. Reluctantly, I let them take over completely; after all, they knew exactly what they were doing. I remember thinking this must dreadful for this child, no-one ever thinks what the baby is going through. One minute it is sitting in all this lovely liquid and the next it is squeezed into a dark tunnel it can't get out of.

Then it was like something out of a horror movie. These dreadful stirrups arrived and and it was like being in a nightmare. I didn't feel like me any more; it was as if I was just a vagina and no other part of me existed. The guiding light in all of this was the anaesthetist and I really grabbed on to him.

He talked to me while everyone else was busy with my other end, and explained that he was going to give me a spinal block which would numb me from the waist down and work extremely quickly. I thought, 'Oh God, it's an injection, Phil hates them'. So we decided it would be better if he waited outside!

I rolled over, the anaesthetist injected me, and within seconds it worked. I don't know why they don't do it all the time because it was wonderful. From then on I was aware of my body being manipulated but felt nothing.

Phil came back and luckily I didn't see what came next. Apparently they wedged this great steel contraption in between my legs and inserted something to open the cervix so they could get the forceps in. I just heard this cranking noise as they opened me up. I couldn't feel it, but Phil's eyes were watering for me!

From the moment the baby's heartbeat had dropped until now had literally taken only about five minutes and suddenly it was all over. They waited for me to have a contraction and then, as I pushed, they lifted her out and I had this wonderful sensation of my body vacating. She was covered in all this grease and gunge but I thought she was the most beautiful thing I had ever seen.

The rest of the room just seemed to recede until it didn't exist; there was just this little sort of cave with Phillip, Laura and myself inside. It felt really wonderful, the strongest sensation I've ever had in my life.

Chin, 40, hospital sister, and Alan, 44, surveyor

"This one's done a flip, we've got a breech here"

"It felt like a knife had been rammed into me"

"You've got two here!"

After the birth of my son, Paul, seven years ago, I discovered I had endometriosis. This is when the lining of the uterus travels out through the fallopian tubes into the abdominal cavity and eventually forms blood-filled cysts. Unfortunately this can lead to infertility and, although I had corrective surgery, I still didn't fall pregnant after many years of trying. In the end we looked at the other options open to us and were lucky to be accepted on to an IVF programme.

IVF stands for In Vitro Fertilization, a process by which eggs are collected using a laparoscopy, usually done under general anaesthetic, and then fertilized in a test tube with your partner's sperm. The eggs are checked over the next 48 hours and, if fertilization is achieved, the resulting embryos are introduced directly into the womb. With me, 18 eggs were collected and I think the average is about six, so I was very lucky.

The following day four embryos were put back inside me but unfortunately they didn't take. When our second attempt failed, Alan said, "That's enough, no more". He felt that the stress of failure was too much for me, and although I agreed to stop the programme, mentally I had prepared myself. After all, it was just like trying for a baby in normal circumstances and that doesn't always happen straightaway either.

I still longed for another child and we decided to try for adoption. Understandably, this is a very long process and, although we were accepted as prospective parents, I couldn't take my mind off the remaining embryos at the IVF clinic. Alan was still against the idea, he couldn't understand the desire within me to have another baby, the urge to carry on until I had one.

I became very depressed at this point and finally ended up in my local church praying for some guidance. Each time I prayed I was led back to the embryos, so that in the end I said to Paul, "Look I can't stop thinking about them, they're there and I can't ignore them any longer". So I went ahead and rang the clinic.

One month later I was pregnant. I just couldn't believe it: after all the years of waiting, finally I was expecting a baby. I told Alan immediately. He was completely taken aback, but just as excited as I was, and for the rest of the week we were both on cloud nine. After the initial euphoria I tried to bring myself back down to earth, because the percentage of women on the programme who lose their babies is quite high, and I realised that this was just the beginning. I had to learn to accept that this was only a pregnancy and that there were plenty of things that could still go wrong.

The other worry I had was whether or not to have an amniocentesis. I was 40 at the time and I knew that the question would be raised sooner or later. I wasn't keen – there is a risk of spontaneous abortion and the pregnancy was vulnerable as it was. I discussed it at length with my GP and, as I had suspected, he was very keen for me to go through with the test.

He pointed out that when the child reached 30, I would be 70 and if it was a Down's syndrome baby, there would be no way I could cope. Of course, everything he said made complete sense, so I came away not knowing what to do. In the end Alan said, "Look Chin, you are not going to abort even if you find out it is a Down's baby are you?" I realised at that moment that of course I wasn't, so that was that.

At eight weeks I went to the hospital for my first scan. I'll never forget the look on the doctor's face as she examined the screen; her eyes just widened and she said, "You've got two here!" My initial reaction was a mixture of great happiness and total panic. I turned to my husband, who had gone as white as a sheet, and said, "Oh Lord, *two* !"

It took a bit of time, but we soon got used to the idea and from then on I just sailed through. I was very sensible with my diet and took as much rest as possible. I was definitely aware of two babies being inside me. One was to the right and very active the whole time, while the other one on the left was much quieter and more peaceful.

By the end, I was bordering on the gigantic and there wasn't much room left in an Evans size 24! Sometimes I was very proud that I had this huge tummy and other times it was just… ahhhgh! I worried that I wouldn't be able to shift the weight once the babies were born, but a friend who had twins herself reassured me that you do so much running around it soon all comes off.

Having already had one child, I didn't have any false expectations about what the birth would be like. With twins anything can happen and you have to be as open-minded as possible. I fully expected to have an epidural, I knew it would hurt and I didn't want to be a martyr; plus if I found myself in the situation where a Caesarean became unavoidable, at least I would be awake throughout the procedure.

At 35 weeks my waters broke in the middle of the night. It was like a flood, literally. I stood up and it just poured and poured until the whole place was awash. Alan carted Paul off to a friend who was on standby, while I took a shower. I wasn't having any contractions and was actually quite calm. When Alan got back we rang the hospital and they said to come in fairly promptly and we left about 4am.

When we arrived they wired me up to a monitor and after about two hours it began to register quite strong contractions. I was beginning to feel them for myself and asked for a Tens machine. We walked around for a while, which seemed to help, but as the labour progressed I asked for the epidural. I wasn't in excruciating pain but wanted it in before that happened and I was still in control.

I asked them not to give me a full wack, so that I wouldn't be totally numb and would still have the sensation to push. Things seemed to move quite slowly after that. I was aware of my contractions, but not in any pain. Everybody was chatting away and I felt relaxed and happy. It was an exciting time.

Around mid-day the midwife examined me and said I was fully dilated. 'Oh great', I thought, now we can get going. Soon I'd be holding the babies I had longed for. I started to push and push, I put all my strength into it but nothing happened. The midwife encouraged me: "Come on now, you can do it, try again". So off I went, push, push, push. I pushed like crazy and still nothing, no movement from either baby; what was going on? Finally, a consultant was called.

He did a quick internal examination and announced that the first baby was posterior, which meant that the head was lying in the wrong position for a normal delivery and that I would have to have forceps. I can't tell you how cross I was. All those hours of pushing had been for nothing. Surely the midwife should have known there was a problem and acted much sooner.

I was transferred to the operating theatre in case a Caesarean was necessary. I think they were worried that the babies were getting distressed, I know I was. The consultant explained that they would increase the epidural dose to numb the entire area, but as it would take at least ten minutes to travel down he was also going to give me a local anaesthetic. Oh boy, did that sting.

It was, however, nothing compared to the forceps going in, the pain took my breath away. It felt like a knife had been rammed in to me. I begged them for more pain relief and they handed me the gas and air. I breathed in enormous lungsful, gulp after gulp, anything to ease the pain.

I was beginning to lose all awareness when suddenly I was presented with my first baby girl. I just had a glimpse of her before they whisked her off. I didn't feel any emotion, it was almost as if I was an outsider, completely detached from what was going on. I vaguely heard the consultant saying, "This one's done a flip, we've got a breech here". I didn't feel any more pain, but seemed to drift in and out of consciousness. The next thing I remember is Alan saying, "Look Chin, we've got another little girl".

I desperately wanted to hold her, but felt too weak and was scared I'd drop her. Both babies were taken to the special care unit. We were told that this was just a precautionary measure, because although they were perfectly healthy with good weights (5lb 10oz and 5lb 7oz), they were still five weeks premature.

They progressed very quickly in special care and it was only a week before we were allowed to bring them home. It was wonderful finally to walk through my front door with not just one, but two, beautiful healthy baby girls. I'd waited years for this moment. I sat down on the sofa and put them both to my breast. My little son Paul was kneeling at my feet and as I looked at each of their faces in turn my eyes filled with tears of joy.

Jane, 28, feature writer, and Mark, 30, graphic designer

"I bet you're glad you're a man"

"I'd find myself wondering if the bin in the corner was large enough to throw my breakfast up into"

"The confirmation hit me like a ton of bricks and I totally freaked out"

My pregnancy wasn't entirely planned – well it wasn't planned at all really. We were on holiday and too much wine, hot sun and lazing around in bed led to one slip-up too many, and Bob's your uncle… When at first I didn't get a period I tried to ignore it, but as the weeks passed I had to face up to the inevitable. The confirmation hit me like a ton of bricks and I totally freaked out. What were we going to do?

Mark and I had never really discussed having children. We assumed that we'd have them one day but we had so many other plans that a baby just didn't enter into the picture at that moment in our lives. We certainly weren't set up for it either, we only lived in a one bedroom flat and the anticipated loss of one income wouldn't exactly put us in a financial position to buy a bigger place.

I was just at a point where my career was progressing quite nicely. I was working for the magazine *Design Week* and loved what I was doing and, of course, although you think you can go back to work, the logistics don't always work out. It's easy to say, 'Oooh, a lovely baby, everything's going to be wonderful and we'll work it out somehow' but that's a very idealistic attitude. I wasn't ready for this baby, and I knew it.

Mark and I sat down and discussed what we were going to do and, although it had briefly gone through our minds, we both knew that a termination was out of the question. We decided not to tell anybody straight away, firstly because we needed to get our own heads around it and secondly, as Mark pointed out, anything can go wrong in the first three months. I suppose I just let the days drift by and didn't face up to what was happening. It wasn't until I began to feel the physical effects of the pregnancy that things really hit home.

We still hadn't told anyone and, believe you me, it's very difficult keeping up the pretence of normality when your hormones are going doolally. I got the most awful morning sickness, which is not very conducive to a good day's work. I'd find myself wondering if the bin in the corner was big enough to throw my breakfast up into. Also because no-one knew, I didn't get the support and encouragement that I guess I needed. I began to feel increasingly alone and isolated. I wanted to ask masses of questions and in the end I made an appointment at the Brook Advisory Centre in London. I knew they dealt primarily with terminations, but went anyway in the hope that they might have some information for me. They couldn't really help, although they did give me the number of the National Childbirth Trust. I tried it a few times, but there was always an answering machine on so I gave up in the end.

I didn't find my GP much help either: my appointment was so rushed that there wasn't enough time to ask any questions, and I just had the normal tests and out I went. My morning sickness was still terrible and then I read a book about homoeopathy and how effective it can be in alleviating symptoms.

I made an appointment at a clinic and although it was very expensive it was certainly worth it. I was there for ages and she really spent a lot of time talking to me about my fears and the problems I was facing. I can't say the remedy she gave me completely eradicated the sickness, but it definitely helped.

About this time, I started telling people that I was pregnant and found that finally being able to acknowledge it was a step in the right direction. I carried on working, and as I got bigger and bigger I found it a bit of a strain. It was a long trek in and out every day, I hated those journeys. When you're squashed up on a commuter train and no-one will give you a seat all you want to do is be at home with a cup of tea and your feet up. I eventually left work at the end of January and my baby was due on either the 1st or 18th April; no-one was quite sure, least of all me.

After wanting to leave work for so long, I suddenly found myself at home and completely at a loss as to what to do. I had no structure to the day and would wake up after Mark had gone to work, feeling completely alone. I became very anxious, it seemed that the situation could only get worse because soon I would have a baby to look after and then there really would be no escape. I think a lot of my problems stemmed from the fact that all my friends and family lived quite a long way away and I just didn't know anybody in the area.

The turning point for me came when on one of my check-ups I met Dorothy, a wonderful midwife who ran antenatal swimming classes. Suddenly I was surrounded by lots of other pregnant women and after each session we'd sit around nattering for ages over a cup of tea and a sticky bun. Dorothy did her best to allay all our fears with comments like, "What are you worried about? Women have been having babies for thousands of years, it's what we do".

Although this helped, I have to say I was still pretty much blocking out the big day. As a consequence, I didn't sort out my birth plan, thinking I'd cross all those bridges when I came to them. I did consider that I'd quite like not to have painkillers but on the other hand I knew if I needed them I'd have them!

Towards the end, I was getting enormous. I began to worry because I'm only 4ft 11 and the bulge seemed to protrude almost to the same proportions. I voiced my concern to the consultant at the hospital, and he very condescendingly said, "Don't worry Miss Lewis, small mothers give birth to small babies, you'll be fine". I wouldn't have been surprised if he'd patted me on the head and sent me off with a lollipop. Actually, that was fairly indicative of how I was treated whenever I went to the hospital.

By the time my first due date arrived, 1st April, I was very, very uncomfortable. I had enormous pressure on my bladder and pelvic area, which made walking virtually impossible. I wasn't sleeping and, to cap it all, I'd trapped a nerve in my back which was so painful that, on my doctor's advice, I was taking up to eight Paracetamol a day. I was longing for the birth now – ironic really, when it had been the one thing I'd been dreading most of all. Like everything, it happened when I least expected it.

I was on the phone to my friend at about 9.30pm when suddenly my waters went. It felt like I was weeing myself and I remember thinking, 'Thank God I've got up off the new sofa'. I dropped the phone, leaving my friend just hanging at the other end, and shot into the loo. I yelled to Mark in a real panic, "Ring the hospital!" and they told us to come in right away.

We were both fumbling around like a pair of idiots, trying to remember all the things we needed. As we drove to the hospital I tried to stay calm and not get myself too worked up.

I wasn't given an internal because, as my waters had broken, they were worried about the risk of infection. They wanted to check out the baby's heartbeat so I was strapped up to a monitor. At first the reading was very slow and they explained that the baby was sleeping and they would have to wake it up to get an active heartbeat.

They did this by manipulating my bump, which I found really quite uncomfortable. It took ages, but finally they got a response and I was relieved to hear that everything was okay. I was told that although my waters had broken I wasn't actually in labour yet and therefore it was best that Mark went home so that I could get some sleep on the ward. I went to bed feeling really scared because Mark wasn't there; everything was dark and it was such a horrible situation to be in. They'd given me some painkillers and sleeping tablets, neither of which seemed to have any effect. I couldn't sleep because I was getting very strong contractions. They weren't regular but they were painful, and I found it very upsetting to be told by the night nurse that I wasn't in proper labour and to go back to sleep.

By morning they were much worse; I was grimacing and clenching my fists. It was a cramping kind of pain with lots of lower backache and this terrible pressure bearing down. By 10 o'clock they were coming every 15 minutes. As my waters were still leaking out I had to wear a big bulky sanitary towel and when I went to the loo I discovered a greenish stain. One of the midwives told me this was meconium and then things began to really hot up. They were concerned that some of the meconium might have got into the baby's lungs and, as I wasn't even dilating yet, they felt it best to induce me.

Mark arrived and we were taken to the delivery suite. I was instantly wired up to a drip and got into a bit of a panic. I didn't want it to happen like this, I felt rushed and very shaky. The contractions had slowed down but I could still feel things happening; they were very irregular but quite painful and I was trying to breathe through them. I was handling things okay at this stage and had calmed down a bit from the initial shock of discovering the meconium and being induced. Two doctors walked in and, after examining me, they discovered that even though I had been induced I still wasn't dilating. They bluntly told me that if I didn't dilate 2cms within the next two hours, I'd have to have a Caesarean.

I couldn't believe it. "Why me?" My heart started pounding and a wave of fear crept over me, starting from my toes and welling up throughout my entire body. I started crying, I didn't want a Caesarean, how was I supposed to make my body dilate if it wasn't ready to? The midwives did their best to console me, but I was still very frightened. It was mid-day. I remember looking at the clock and thinking how the hell am I going to get through the next two hours; I was totally out of control.

The contractions started to get stronger and stronger; I'd lost my rhythm with the breathing and went on to the gas and air, but in all honesty, I was so freaked out, I knew I wasn't using it properly. Mark could see how distressed I was and suggested I have an epidural. I'd been so out of it that it hadn't occurred to me and instantly I said, "Yes". It made so much sense, if I was going to have a Caesarean at least I would be awake for the birth and hopefully it would ease things enough for me to get a grip on the situation.

As we waited for the anaesthetist to arrive, they asked if I minded a trainee midwife giving me an internal examination. This was like a red rag to a bull; I couldn't trust myself to speak, and luckily Mark very politely said he didn't think it was a good idea. By the time I had the epidural, the contractions were coming every three to five minutes and were awful, but it took very quickly. The effect was amazing, I couldn't feel any pain at all and it was the best thing for me, because it helped to calm me down, although not completely.

I was still scared about the threat of a Caesarean hanging over me and on the dot of two the doctors walked back in. By this point I'd turned them into two monsters, to me they were like the bloody gestapo. In their brusque, dominating manner I was informed that God must be looking down on me as I had dilated the required amount, but I wasn't to count my chickens because I was given the same criteria for the next two hours. I remember lying there thinking, 'I can't believe you're letting yourself go through this'. It was just so awful. I turned to Mark and said, "I bet you're glad you're a man!"

I carried on dilating fairly slowly until, eventually, at around 6pm, I was told the heat was off. Apparently they now seemed confident that my body was responding in the way they saw fit and a Caesarean wouldn't be necessary. I was tremendously relieved, but still really unhappy with the situation; the hospital seemed to be controlling me every step of the way and I didn't feel strong enough to argue with them. The epidural slowly began to wear off and I could feel the pain coming back again.

During the next few hours I seemed to cope a lot better. Mark was holding my hand and together we were breathing through the contractions. I can't say I was enjoying myself, but at least I felt a little in control. Then, at 9.30, the consultant arrived and out of the blue said, "It's time to get this baby out, we'll do a forceps delivery!" I started to scream inside. For the first time I had been controlling my labour and now they wanted to take it away from me again.

I yelled at him, "No, I'm starting to get into it, I want to push the baby out myself". He tried to reason with me and explained that it was hospital policy to deliver babies as quickly as possible after 24 hours of labour, "Because the mother may get overtired and, also, the babies are often distressed by this stage, and we don't want that to happen". So that was that.

My legs were put into stirrups, which for me was one of the most uncomfortable parts of all. My knees were pushed up against my bump and I felt totally vulnerable and at their mercy. The fear began to rise again and then I became aware of the doctor saying, "This is a big baby, why has no-one told me this before? We're dealing with at least a nine-pounder here". I totally flipped out; as I said, I'm only 4ft 11, how the hell were they going to get it out? The epidural had almost worn off completely and I felt it as he cut me, although I must say it didn't really hurt; I was just aware of something going on in that region.

The forceps were in place and I was told to push. I was screaming with the effort, it wasn't agonizingly painful, just unbearably uncomfortable. He was pulling and I was pushing. I put everything I had into it, I just wanted the baby out. Mark was behind me saying, "Come on, Jane, you can do it!" I filled my lungs and pushed with all my might and eventually they pulled her out of me. I started to shake all over; I was saying, "I'm so cold, please cover me". I'd lost a lot of blood, and one of the nurses was saying, "She's in shock". I was so frightened for myself I didn't care what was going on with the baby. I vaguely remember Mark holding the baby and showing her to me. I

112

don't remember any immediate feelings of love, I was just out of it completely, it was as if I wasn't there. I could hear her crying for what seemed like ages – she didn't like being born like that and I didn't like it either. It was all kisses and congratulations, but I felt really ill, like I had food poisoning or flu or something. We were taken back to the ward and Rosie was taken to the nursery. I was so shattered that I fell asleep the moment my head hit the pillow.

I woke up in the middle of the night, startled to think, 'Oh, my God I've got a baby, I must be responsible now', but physically I didn't have the strength to do anything.

The next day I felt a little better, but very apathetic. I went to collect Rosie from the nursery but although I had intended to breast-feed her I just couldn't bring myself to do it. The following day I did put her to the breast and I suppose that was the beginning of the bonding process.

Rosie had been a shock to me from the moment I conceived her. My whole world had been turned upside down. But I did fall in love, totally and utterly, and now I could never be without her.

WHAT THE MEN SAID...

The baby's head was delivered face down and with one swift movement the midwife turned it face up. I honestly thought, 'They've killed my baby, they've broken its neck'. I was just about to pounce when the little thing opened its mouth and let out an almighty wail. The midwife looked up at me and said, "Healthy pair of lungs". Six months on I can confirm she was right on target with that comment.

Sarah was swearing like a trooper. Every time I touched her she mouthed some obscenity at me which basically meant, 'Leave me alone'. I felt totally useless, completely out of my depth. I'd been to all the classes and read all the books but the actual event was nothing like it.

Seeing the baby come out was tremendously exciting. I felt dizzy with euphoria.

It was nothing like I imagined it would be. Watching someone you love in that much pain and not being able to help is terrible. When Sally had the epidural I felt much more relaxed, suddenly she was normal again. The actual delivery was incredible, there isn't anything quite like it. It was a very special moment.

I have to say it, cliche or not, I'm extremely glad I'm not a woman.

I couldn't handle it at all. I spent most of the time in the corridor outside. Whenever I went back into the room I felt sick. I feel as if I let Carrie down, I just wasn't there when she needed me.

You women definitely change when you're pregnant. My wife was so irritable, nothing I did was right. I remember once coming home with a bunch of flowers hoping to cheer her up, and she burst into tears yelling at me that she wasn't an invalid. The birth was a doddle by comparison.

There's no point asking me. I nipped out for a cup of tea and missed the whole thing.

Charlie was born by Caesarean section which both of us found quite traumatic. It all became very medical and serious. Like any new experience you're just not sure what to do for the best.

Janet says she couldn't have done it without me but to be honest it was a bit like the blind leading the blind.

I just couldn't come to terms with seeing my wife with her legs wide open being prodded and poked about by male doctors. I really had to control the urge to leap up and pull them off her.

I was so proud of Rosie. We had both wanted the birth to be as natural as possible. I did all I could to encourage her, helping with the breathing and rubbing her back. We were both focused on the task together, it was such a 'human' experience. The depth of feeling between us and then little Briony was overwhelming.

Communication is what it's all about. Everyone involved has different ideas. I'd say one thing, she'd say something else and the delivery team would have yet another idea. To sum it up, confusing.

I wouldn't have missed it for the world. I feel sorry for those fathers who have never experienced it. It certainly brings you closer together.

I was scared stiff. I thought, 'I've done this to her, I've put her in this situation'. I wanted it to be over but it just went on for hours – 18 in the end. I'd certainly want to be better prepared next time round.

She was gripping my hand so hard I thought she was going to break it. I was amazed she had that much strength. All credit to her though, from my side of the bed it looked like bloody hard work.

I was useless in the delivery room. I should have been around in the days when they paced about outside.

Hillary was fabulous, she was totally calm and relaxed, I was in awe of her. I found myself responding instantly to her every command. When Joshua was born she handed him up to me and said, "Happy Fatherhood". My eyes still fill up whenever I think about it.

It was brilliant, absolutely brilliant. I fell in love with my wife all over again.

GLOSSARY

Amniocentesis
A technique of removing fluid from the amniotic sac surrounding a foetus in order to detect certain genetic disorders and birth defects including Down's syndrome (Mongolism) and Tay-Sachs disease

Braxtons Hicks contractions
Irregular contractions of the muscles of the uterus that occur throughout pregnancy

Breech Birth
When the baby presents itself buttocks first

Caesarean Section
Delivery of a baby through a surgical incision in the uterus

Dilation
This is when the cervix opens out fully (normally 10cms) to allow the baby's head to pass through

Effacement of the Cervix
Before the cervix can dilate it must be thinned and softened; this process is called effacement

Electronic Foetal Monitoring
This is a method of recording a baby's heartbeat and the mother's contractions during labour

Epidural
A regional anaesthesia that is administered by injection into a space between the ligaments of the bony vertebrae in the mother's back, thereby deadening pain from the abdominal area down

Episiotomy
An incision made in the perineum (between the vaginal opening and the anus) to enable easier delivery of the baby and to prevent tearing

Forceps Delivery
A two-bladed instrument, resembling a pair of tongs, that is used to extract a baby

Gas and Air
A combination of nitrous oxide and trilene which is self-administered through a mask

Internal examination
In pregnancy: To confirm the pregnancy and to check that the uterus is the size it should be according to date. To check for pelvic abnormalities and that the cervix is tightly closed
In labour: To establish rate of effacement and dilation

Meconium
The presence of Meconium in the amniotic fluid indicates that the baby has had a bowel movement and could be in distress

Obstetrician
A doctor who specialises in childbirth including antenatal and postnatal care

Pre-eclampsia
A condition that develops in the last trimester of pregnancy. Symptoms include high blood pressure, protein in the urine and fluid retention

Show
The appearance of the blood-tinged plug of mucus that has blocked the cervical canal during pregnancy

Ultrasound Scan
A photographic picture which is formed by the echoes and soundwaves bouncing off different parts of the body. Unlike X-rays, ultrasound can record soft tissue in detail and will print out a highly accurate picture of the foetus

Ventouse Extraction
A small metal cup which is connected to a vacuum appartus is passed
into the vagina and applied to the baby's head. A vacuum is created,
the cup sticks to the baby's scalp and by gentle pulling, and the mother
pushing, the baby is delivered

Waters, rupture of
This is when the amniotic fluid surrounding the baby breaks during
labour and gushes or leaks out of the vagina

HELPLINES

Active Birth Movement,
55 Dartmouth Park Road,
London NW5 1SL
Tel: 071 267 3006
Offers support and advice to women who want to try and have a
natural childbirth. Rents collapsible birth pools

Association of Radical Midwives,
62 Greetsby Hill,
Ormskirk,
Lancs L39 2DT
Tel: 0695 72776 or 071 580 2991
May be able to put you in touch with an independent midwife in your
area

Baby Soother Tapes,
JayGee Cassettes,
10 Golf Links Road,
Burnham-on-Sea,
Somerset TA8 2PW

Birthworks,
4e Brentmill Estate,
South Brent,
Devon, TQ1 09YT
Tel: 0364 72802
Hires out collapsible, portable birthing pools

Caesarean Support Network,
2 Hurst Park Drive,
Huyton,
Liverpool L36 1TF
Tel: 051 480 1184
Support from a contacts network at meetings or over the telephone

Gingerbread,
35 Wellington Street,
London WC2E 7BN
Tel: 071 240 0953
Offers help and support for single parent families

Multiple Births Foundation,
Institute of Obstetrics and Gynaecology,
Queen Charlotte's and Chelsea Hospital,
Goldhawk Road,
London W6 0XG
Tel: 081 748 4666
Offers help and support to mothers of twin, triplet, quad or higher
order births

Pre-eclampsic Toxaemia Society,
33 Keswick Avenue,
Hullbridge,
Essex SS5 6JZ
Tel: 0702 231689
Offers advice and support and possible avoidance tactics

Mama (Meet a Mum Association),
58 Malden Avenue,
London SE25 4HS
Tel: 081 656 7318
Help to all new mothers, but particularly those suffering from
postnatal depression

NEEN Pain Management Systems (Tens),
Old Pharmacy Yard,
Church Street,
Deveham,
Norfolk NR19 1DJ
Tel: 0362 698966
Hire of Tens machines

Nippers,
C/o The Sam Segal Perinatal Research Unit,
St Mary's Hospital,
Praed Street,
Paddington,
London W2 1NY
Tel: 071 725 1487
Information for parents of premature babies

West London Birth Centre,
St Stephens Road,
Ealing,
London, W13 8HB
Tel: 081 998 0548
Offers pre- and postnatal yoga classes. Information on yoga in all
areas

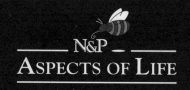

N&P
ASPECTS OF LIFE

Aspects of Life is a series of publications designed to help people respond to the changing circumstances which they face as their lives progress.

In an entertaining and down-to-earth style, the Aspects of Life Series seeks to encourage readers not only to tackle their responsibilities in a more fulfilling way, but also to enjoy the stimulus of new challenges.

The subject matter, which at present ranges through home life, leisure and work, is being chosen to recognise the diversity of experience and opportunities which individuals and families may encounter.

This pioneering venture by a building society draws on N&P's unique experience in responding to customers' requirements, helping people to achieve a better quality of life.